HEARTFUSION
THE MAGIC OF IMPRINTING WATER

HeartFusion™

The Magic of Imprinting Water

By

Jana Shiloh, MA, CCH

Life Resources Publishing
Sedona, AZ

First Edition

Designer: Jana Shiloh, MA, CCH

Cover Art: Linda Bruce. www.lindabruceart.com

Acknowledgments

This book is dedicated, in memoriam, to Dr. George Graff who first introduced me to homeopathy, and Mr. Babaji who has guided me all along the way.

A special thanks to: George Vithoulkas, Vega Rozenberg, Ram Das AKA Dr. Richard Alpert, Dr. Rajan Shankaran, Dr. Devin Mikles, Dr. Ashok Gangadeen, Clayton Nolte, Donna Anderson, Franz Herbst, Dr. Emoto, and to so many close friends and mentors too numerous to mention. And thank you to Linda Bruce for the wonderful cover art.

Endorsements for the Book

"Jana Shiloh has developed an amazing technology to quickly shift a person from a stressful and incoherent experience into a state of coherence and balance. I personally experienced her simple and efficient approach, while monitoring myself with the em-Wave desktop (from the Institute of HeartMath) and I immediately achieved a state of coherence and inner peace after using my custom made HeartFusion™ essence. I highly recommend this book."

Dr. Annette Deyhle, PhD, Research Coordinator, Institute of HeartMath, Boulder Creek, CA

"The author offers the reader a surprisingly simple yet profoundly exciting method for healing your emotions, mind, and body by instantly creating new pathways in your brain.

Jana Shiloh reveals her own lifelong journey as a spiritual seeker, human being, and homeopathic practitioner, She summarizes the concepts of homeopathy, structured water, and the research of Dr. Emoto, to show that everything is energy and frequency. Integrating these concepts with her life, and clinical experience, she has created a new modality- "Heartfusion™." This clinically tested process, using imprinted water, is an amazingly powerful self-help method for anyone wishing to heal and dramatically change their life. It focuses on dissolving core issues and emotions that affect the patterns in our lives, as well as our bodies, minds and spirit.

The book is interesting and well written with succinct testimonials and clear instructions. You will enjoy this lively account. I recommend it highly for anyone who wants to grow and heal."

Dr. Jessie J. Mercay, PhD, PhDmsta (former wholistic health practitioner and current Chancellor of the American University of Mayonic Science and Technology)

"In her new book, *The Magic of Imprinting Water*, Jana Shiloh, a homeopathic educator with several decades of experience, dedicated study and research, gives us a glimpse of her own path towards mastery of the homeopathic method. This process has given birth to a new and advanced homeopathic tool which anyone can make for themselves. It sparks the body's own innate healing system into activity. Jana has a knack for healing, comforting, inspiring and transforming that stands as an excellent example for all of us on the path of healing. Her innovative approaches in homeopathy, her integrity, persistence, and creativity, are a light to those of us who aspire to understand natural healing. I have personally experienced the magic of creating a HeartFusion™. I enthusiastically encourage you to try this process for yourself."

Dr. Devin A. Mikles, MD, MD(H), FACP

Table of Contents

Introduction

Putting the Power into Your Hands:
Transformation Made Easy

I ask you a critical question: What is more important to you than anything else in the world? Is it your family? Your pet? Your spouse? Your best friend? Your work? Success? Spiritual development? What is your bottom line in life?

Consider that the bottom line is you! If you are irritable, flare up in anger, are always depressed, in grief, or out of emotional balance in any way, can you be available to your loved ones? For the passions in life? What could you create? What could you actually do? The real bottom line is: how limited are you? What gets in your way of enjoyment? What changes *in you* would allow you to be a healthier, happier person? What changes would make your life easier? More exciting?

Have you ever had severe physical or emotional pain? If you've been living on this planet, chances are the answer is yes. Sometimes we can find relief--the kind of relief drugs give, like painkillers, and mood-altering drugs, alcohol, and for some, street drugs. But where can we find a *real* answer? An answer that gets to the root of the matter? Something that actually cures, as opposed to temporarily covering up the problem? Often when pain is not responsive to the usual methods of treatment (or even the unusual!) it may mean the pain has its roots deep in the emotions where drugs, herbs, exercise, and other alternative methods cannot always reach. I learned this the hard way...after a bout of six months of sciatic pain. Using this new process I discovered, the pain got resolved in an unusual way.

We know the mind and emotions have powerful effects on our bodies and our lives; we have learned about how important it is to change our minds, our emotions, our belief systems and more. We have read self-help books, and watched a DVD with Oprah about "The Secret." But who is giving us methods to really do this in a deep, effective way, a way that can actually transform the underlying energetic patterns that give rise to our emotions and our chemistry? We need to be able to effect a *real* transformation, even into the neuropathways of our brains, thereby affecting us on *all* levels. There are many techniques out there, but most will basically tell you to change, think positively, and feel the corresponding emotions with those thoughts. There is evidence that our emotions have a powerful effect on our chemistry, and sometimes *vice versa!* We need a simple method that will support us every time and bring a deep, immediate shift, not just touching the mental mind, but the deep energetic imprint underlying everything else. We need a method that unravels the patterns that bind us.

I believe I have found one answer; it is powerful and simple once understood. It is a process that you can learn in an in-depth private session, a workshop, or through this book. It can be used when needed, allowing you to instantly change feeling and perception, your brain chemistry in a blink of the eye! It always works if you follow directions. Everything I am about to share with you has been tested and proven not only on my own 'body/mind," but on many others, both in workshops and in private sessions.

As I said, I myself have had an on-and-off history of sciatic pain. In my last episode, I tried all my usual homeopathic remedies that had worked in the past, but to no avail. I tried all forms of treatment (I have lots of friends in the healing profession) but nothing worked. I spent a terrible summer in constant pain, unable to be comfortable sitting, walking or lying, mostly stuck in my home. Finally one day I decided to try my new method for emotional transformation on my own body, using the technique I will share in this book. I had made a HeartFusion™ for a core issue of mine a few months earlier, but I decided to make it stronger. I began to use it directly on my lower back. To my amazement, the pain began to melt away! In two days I was pain free. This was the first time I had full relief in seven months! Now, on rare occasions, if I get twinges of pain from sitting too long in an uncomfortable chair, I will use it again, and the pain dissolves. This even after I was told by a physical therapist I had a disc problem! I was already in the process of writing this book when I discovered this self-made remedy affected not only my emotions but also my physical body in a way I had not expected. Now, I am even more motivated to share this amazing discovery with you. It's easy, and once learned, you can make your own in your kitchen!

We seem to be entering a time of increased suppression in the world of medicine. Homeopathy and all forms of alternative medicine are again under attack, just when those gifts are more important than ever. While writing it was tempting to make this into a research project to prove homeopathy works, as homeopathic principles are part of this process. Although I have felt it necessary to put some relevant research and information into this book, it is not my purpose to try to prove homeopathy to the skeptics in science (which has already been attempted many times over). I am only interested in educating people with common sense and an open mind. The premises of homeopathy are extremely important but have been ignored and ridiculed by much of the American scientific community since the early 1900s. This has not been true in other countries.

I would ask you to read this book, and try these discoveries for yourself with an open mind. *You* be the judge! It is written for you! Only then will you know the truth!

Those who have participated privately or in workshops with me have been deeply moved and impressed with the results. Without personal experience, this whole thing is reduced to mental gymnastics as to who is right and who is wrong, "Does it work or doesn't it? Is it real or imaginary?" Over my 30 years in homeopathy, I have repeatedly seen the powerful effects of homeopathy. In addition, I have seen the amazing, instantaneous results of this new method over and over again in all age groups and situations. From the time I was really young, it was my deepest desire to discover something that would help humanity. I am happy and honored to introduce you to this expansion of homeopathic principles; this system empowers everyone to transform emotional and physical imbalances. I thank all of my teachers on all levels for providing me with the many pieces to this puzzle. Since homeopathic principles, and the process of making a homeopathic remedy, are at the foundation of this new method, I will be discussing homeopathy in depth at first, and sharing some of its secrets! It is important that you understand it, among other things, so as to appreciate the process. This is an autobiographical, educational, self-help book!

This adventure all started almost 30 years ago when I first learned of the profound healing effects of homeopathy. I was treated by a homeopath when my life was in shambles. Because of homeopathy, my sanity returned naturally, quickly, mysteriously, and incomprehensively, without the use of drugs. I became calm and found myself again. Because of my deep gratitude, homeopathy has become my all-consuming passion ever since. Over the years I have seen many miracles and cures with friends and clients; there was also the moment when it saved my former husband's life!

I am here to tell a fascinating story--one that I can see, in retrospect, has been revealed like a treasure hunt over many years. It culminated in a discovery that amazed me: the curing of my sciatic pain along with the shifting of a deep core issue. The exciting information I am about to relate can open amazing doors for all of us. You can be a part of these further explorations. I am here to share this with fellow adventurers: those who are open and have ears to hear. I encourage skeptics to do their own real homework. There are many resources listed along the way, as well as at the end of this book where anyone can go to learn more about energy, frequency, homeopathy, and water. In a somewhat unconventional way, I have included many Internet references in the body of the book. I hope you access those sites to learn even more about these subjects.

In the following story you will learn about these "treasures" that I have discovered along with my personal journey, and how all this can transform your life, too. What is life without exploration and adventure? Let this be the beginning of *your* adventure!

I will lay a deeper groundwork so you can accompany me in the thought process that has led to this groundbreaking technique. Otherwise, this process may not make much sense to you, and you might think this whole idea preposterous. The first part requires a deeper knowledge about homeopathy, which I illustrate with some personal experiences. This is a book about concepts, real life, and real experiences that includes some new scientific information along the way.

While I have had profound results myself and with clients using HeartFusion™ remedies, this method should not be considered medical advice, diagnosis or suggestion for treatment of a specific illness.

Chapter 1
In the Beginning...

My Personal Voyage

I had been practicing meditation for five years and had the joy and honor to personally learn from Ram Das, also known as Dr. Richard Alpert, in New Hampshire. After that, for six years I lived in a very intense community of 150 people focused on devotional kundalini yoga, with the powerful teacher whom I loved deeply. I was happy there and had no desire to leave, but in 1981 events conspired to catapult me out and into a new life.

After six years in the spiritual community, my former husband, David, decided to leave. I was torn between following him or staying with my teacher, a way of life, and group of people with whom I was deeply connected. Finally I realized this inner conflict was resulting in a serious break down of my health. The indecision tore at me daily. I would wake up depressed, feeling the grip of the love I had for my husband of 14 years, and the love I had for my chosen way of life. There is an unbearable agony in the heart when one is torn between two people or two paths, especially if they are both loved. The decision seems impossible; yet any action, or non-action, is still a choice for one or the other. I had never been great at making decisions and it seemed there was no resolution to this one. I would often burst into tears at sporadic times of the day, and I cried myself to sleep at night. I couldn't imagine what could await me in the "outside world" that would be as meaningful to me as my life was there. Yet I couldn't imagine being without David either. He was my only family.

If you haven't lived in a subculture like that, you cannot know how difficult it is to leave after a few years of total immersion. No one from the "outside" of such a subculture could possibly understand how big a decision this is. Being in the community was a total commitment. My life there was completely focused on my spiritual development, experiences, and inner connection. The community supported this. More than anything else I wanted the elusive thing called "enlightenment." I had read accounts of yogis who had reached a state of total awareness, seeing energy sparkling everywhere and feeling the presence of God in every moment. I imagined if I stayed in the community long enough something would magically happen, and I would be flooded with a bliss lasting the rest of my life! At least I hoped I would have an awareness of the Presence of the Divine in every moment. I had longed for this shift within me, something that would take me from the mundane to the magnificent! I had not wanted the attachments of children or other distractions and had dedicated my whole life, even prior to the community, to this deep inner search. The spiritual community was the outer fulfillment of this inner longing. I needed to feel and be more than just a person working to keep a roof over my head and food in my mouth. Everything I did there had a larger meaning--even washing a wall! It was done for the whole group, the beloved teacher, and for God.

Some would have called this a cult, but for me that was an irrelevant word. I had "grown up" there. I had learned about unconditional love, about how to live with others, to communicate effectively, and to be strong as an individual instead of depending so much on my husband. Living with others is like being a rock in a tumbler--all of the rough edges get ground off and you have to face things about yourself that you didn't even know were there. In a marriage that is possible, but then you always can just blame the other person for all the wrongs. In a group where everyone sees the same stuff in you, there is no escape. Although it can be extremely painful, if you are committed to growth, in the end you surrender and look at what everyone is telling you. We all had a deep longing for the "Truth," whether painful or blissful: all of us wanted to grow. There was also a deep closeness between us, in part because we lived together, in part because we shared the same passion. This level of intimacy is rarely experienced in our modern day life, even between close friends. I loved the power and depth of connection that was possible with many people who shared my intense desires and passions. If you have not experienced that kind of unity and camaraderie, it is hard to imagine.

Have you ever wondered if there were more to life than what you already know? There is an amazing exhilaration when you discover something that you feel will answer the questions "Why?" or "What is it all about?" Life changes when you find something that gives a new meaning to your life and satisfies that powerful thirst. When I found it, I went into it with all I had. Fortunately, so did my husband. Some never think much about finding that answer, or don't know where to look for it, and give up. There are so many blind alleys that never satisfy. Often we think if we just had a new house, or a car, or a new baby, more money, or even beautiful new clothes, that one or all of those things would make us happy. But somehow those external things never ultimately do it! The ones who are taken with that search are driven to find the answer, plunging forward (sometimes shocking their family and friends) to pursue it. It could be in the arts, music, or science. For me, I found it in a "spiritual path" of meditation, my new teacher, and the community--all of which totally embodied the intensity I craved.

So there I was, six years later, completely submerged in this community. I couldn't decide whether I should leave it or not, even if it were for a short period of time. Yet I did have to decide. Leaving was seen as choosing the profane over God, choosing the mundane over the ultimate chance of enlighten-ment in this life. You were perceived as being either with "them" or against "them:" there was no in-between. Finally, after weeks of silent agony and tears, I decided to go to a psychic. Now understand that this was a major heresy in our community. To go to a mere psychic when you were with our Divine spiritual teacher was unheard of! But I was in such anguish, I felt I needed a neutral third party, and no one else fit the bill. I had seen a psychic only once before. It had been while my father was dying, and that experience had been very helpful.

The Decision

I had heard this psychic was good (not all of them are--and no one is 100% accurate, so ultimately you still have to see what resonates and make your own decisions). As I walked through the door, I saw her sitting at the end of an aisle in a church-like place. She looked up at me and without prompting, before I could even sit down, announced: "You're whole life is about to change!" Her statement startled me. She looked me deep in the eyes and said "you will be moving to the southwest and working with herbs, natural remedies and Native Americans." I sat down, my heart pounding, wondering how she could say all this without giving me a chance to ask her questions. I fumbled, pulling out the two photos I had brought with me, one of my teacher, and one of my husband. After poring over the photos she looked up, said nothing about my teacher, but asked me if I loved my husband. I told her I did. "Then you need to see him within three weeks' time or the door to that relationship will be closed for this lifetime." Suddenly, something clicked inside and a new strength and determination took over as I heard her words. I don't think I would have felt that strength had she said I should stay in the community. I knew in that moment I was going to leave, at least to meet with him, and I vowed to do it within three weeks.

I was teaching stress management courses and in-service training courses to teachers and policemen, and was also doing special classes for the elderly and indigent. It took a lot to finish all the courses earlier than expected, organize my life, buy a used station wagon, pack all of my possessions, and hit the road in less than three weeks! But my course was set and it all seemed right. Suddenly I knew it was *my* life to lead, "right or wrong," "blowing" my enlightenment or not. I needed to get clear about whether I was to be with David, or return to the community and my teacher. Even if I was "spiritually blowing it" by leaving, as I was told, I saw that I had to be true to myself. There was no way to "fool God," if you will. Staying in the community with my teacher, when my heart wasn't totally in it, would never have won me a ticket to enlightenment--even if it were the "right" thing for my soul! But then, who could really know what would be the right thing for my soul?

Immediately after leaving the community I drove to Santa Fe to meet David (we were coming from opposite sides of the country). I drove the 36 hours to Santa Fe with only about eight hours of napping along the way. However the meeting was pretty disastrous. He had already started to see another woman when I had been undecided about leaving the community. At the end of two difficult days he announced his decision to return home. David said, "You could come out to where I am living now, but I cannot promise anything, or how often I would see you." I flared with hurt and anger but said nothing. Walking into the other room I called a friend in Boulder. I used to live with her in the community, and I told her what had happened. She invited me to visit her in Boulder. I knew I needed a break; since I had already left the community, I decided to take more time to be with myself and just BE.

David and I parted, unsure of what the future held for either one of us--apart or together. I jumped into the car, speeding and crying all the way to Boulder, with the torture of the only music on the radio: country western. I was at a loss for what to do, and was too emotional to make a final decision about returning to the community. Instead, I took the opportunity to be on my own for the first time ever, and utilize my meager savings to make a final decision. I was at a crossroads in my life and I knew how important that decision would be... and the words of the psychic were ringing in my ears.

In the end it was neither of the above--not husband or teacher...But that painful indecision and subsequent experience ultimately led me into a greater inner strength, and my new passion: homeopathy.

Chapter 2
Introduction to Homeopathy

Boulder: Meeting Dr. Graff

I knew two people in Boulder, Colorado, who used to live at the community, Jane, and Bob. Bob had a very big house, two kids and needed a part-time nanny for the evenings. He invited me to be with the kids during the week after school, in exchange for which he offered me room and board. I decided it would be a good opportunity to gather myself and take a break from it all. I knew I was in need of finding a healthcare professional in Boulder to support my health, so Jane suggested I go to a chiropractor. She said he also did "something else natural" which she couldn't pronounce.

I arrived at Dr. George Graff's office, knowing nothing about what he did except that I needed an adjustment and help with a potentially serious physical problem. He immediately started asking me about myself. Now at that point I felt like a total basket case (ordinarily I am fairly even emotionally). I was crying morning, noon and especially at night and I couldn't sleep. I was undecided about my life and was devastated at the thought of probably losing my marriage. I had been married since I was barely 20, and David was the one person I had trusted and relied on for 14 years; he had been my best friend and only family. Over time I had lost contact with everyone outside of the community; the people there were the only ones I had been close to for six years. My parents were both dead, and I had no real connection with my distant relatives, except a loose one with a cousin by marriage. I had very little money and felt totally alone and totally scared.

George asked me a lot of questions, I cried the whole time, telling him my whole story. At the end of an hour and a half of telling him everything I could think of about myself, he said, "I have something I think will help you." He disappeared, leaving me to wonder what would help my inner desperation and the deep terror of facing an unknown future, short of a lobotomy! He returned with a few sugar pellets he tossed into my mouth. He also gave me a little box of pellets, and told me to return in two weeks. As an afterthought he adjusted my back and sent me on my way.

I had no idea what had hit me--this whirlwind of one and a half hours of telling my story and answering his questions.... and then I was out on the street, alone again. I felt a mix of grief and anger at David. How could my husband of 14 years not still love me and care about me? How could he just walk away after all we had been through? Inside there was an inner voice that was screaming in fear and emotional pain. It would happen often--I would be just driving along and inside a voice would start screaming and screaming--no words, just screaming...

I had no idea what Dr. Graff had just given me or why. I was certainly not set up for a positive placebo experience. But slowly over the next two weeks things started to change: I started to sleep better, I stopped crying even though my situation had not changed, and I felt I was coming back to "myself." Over time, even the internal screaming subsided.

Upon my return visit to Dr. Graff I felt dramatically more stable in body and mind; inside I had vowed to learn how to do what he did--whatever it was. My father had been a psychologist, and I grew up with that worldview. For me to see this amazing mind/body "bridge" happening with these mysterious little white pills was quite compelling. When I arrived for my return appointment, I told him how much better I was feeling. Then I asked him what those little white pills were. Little did I know that I was about to encounter someone and something that would change my whole life, and the way I viewed life and people, forever.

Dr. George Graff Explains Homeopathy

George took a deep breath and settled into his chair, his clear blue eyes sparkled with excitement. "There is something I want to tell you" he said. "I am studying homeopathy with a world-renowned Greek homeopath, Dr. George Vithoulkas. We are the first group of American doctors to be trained in this 'revival' of a healing modality that was famous in the U.S over 200 years ago. Dr. Samuel Hahnemann, the founder of this system, first researched the principle in 1790. Homeopathy has been accepted all over the world. Even the British Royal Family has a homeopath for their official doctor! In 1900 there were 100 homeopathic hospitals and 20 homeopathic medical schools. In the U.S. perhaps you have heard of 'Hahnemann Hospital' in Philadelphia and 'Flower Fifth Avenue Hospital' in New York?" I nodded. I had grown up in New York City. "Originally, they were both homeopathic hospitals. At that time, it was so accepted that the newly-formed FDA was overseeing and approving the preparation of all homeopathic remedies, which they still do today."

"Later, chemists and 'allopathic' (regular 'western medicine') doctors in this country got together around the early 1900s to get rid of women, blacks, and homeopaths in medicine, and they called themselves the AMA. Previously, during the 1800s, many doctors converted to homeopathy when they saw the miracle cures during the great Cholera, Typhoid, and Scarlet Fever epidemics, as well as the Influenza epidemics of 1918 in the US and Europe. One remedy was so effective it was termed the "Grave Robber" because it literally brought people back from death's door. This is all documented in public health records and writings of the time." [1]

I felt a rush of excitement course through my body as he spoke. There was something that seemed very familiar and important about it, even though I had never heard of the word "homeopathy" until that moment.

George continued and I felt my curiosity rising. "Many famous people--even our presidents--were treated by homeopaths! Even though old man Rockefeller was treated by a homeopath, he still put his money into drug companies because the drugs could be patented, unlike the homeopathic remedies that anyone could make if they knew how. Most of the educated and culturally sophisticated people of the day only used homeopathy. In the end, our Public Health Department logged that in the 1918 flu epidemic, 98% of homeopathic patients were cured, whereas most of the others died." [2]

George went on to explain, "The beauty of homeopathy is that the specially-prepared natural remedies are really energetic; they work on the level of physics, not chemistry. They act simply as a catalyst to stimulate the body's own healing response. The correctly-chosen remedy reflects back to the body the same stuck energetic pattern, or information if you like, of the "disease" or imbalance. This triggers the whole Being, the body/mind or the "Vital Force" (as we call it) into responding to the remedy, and therefore the 'disease.' Our bodies have an amazing healing ability which gets activated all day every day; but sometimes we get stuck in certain areas for many different reasons, and do not heal ourselves."

I was blown away by his enthusiasm. Then he looked steadily at me saying, "I need more help in the office. Would you like to work for me?" I was stunned. He continued "But if you do, you would need to come to the homeopathic classes I am teaching here so you can talk to my patients. Of course you could come for free."

I sat for a moment in shocked silence. Then quietly said, "Thank you" to him, and to Spirit--it was all I could have hoped for and more--an education for free, and a job in Boulder where jobs were so unavailable. My life had just taken its new direction! If I had been trying to create a specific reality for myself, I could not have even envisioned this one, but somehow it was happening anyway! No, I wouldn't be going back to the community, and in the end, not to my husband either. It seemed like it was all destined! Life had found me, and I was in the right flow....

A Little More You Need to Know About
Homeopathy and Why: Some History

This part may seem lengthy, but it will help you understand the process that follows. In going to George's classes, I learned about the history of homeopathy. The founder of modern day homeopathy, Samuel Hahnemann, was a doctor, chemist and linguist (1745-1853). He became disillusioned with the medicine of the time and abandoned it. He accepted a life of great poverty with his family, because in good conscience he couldn't continue with the medicine of his time. He began researching and translating old medical texts in Latin and Greek, looking for a better way. He found the concept of "Let likes be cured by likes" in one of the old Latin texts. This meant that if a poison, for example, could create a group of symptoms in a person, it also had the potential to stimulate a cure of that same grouping of symptoms in a "sick" person (the concept of vaccination originally came from homeopathy). Being an open-minded scientist, he decided to test it on himself.

To make a very long story short, knowing that quinine was an effective cure for malaria, Dr. Hahnemann decided to try it on his own body to see what symptoms it would create. He thought if it would create the symptoms of malaria, it might explain, according to that principle, why it could cure it too. He ingested a lot of the bark of the Cinchoma Tree, which contained quinine. To his surprise, he actually did develop many of the symptoms of malaria! Being a rigorous scientist, he repeated his experiment and consistently found the same results.

Knowing the toxicity of other substances, he started using them in his research. Applying this principle of "The Law of Similars" (let likes be cured by likes, or in Latin: *similia similibus curentur)*, he began to treat illness with diluted amounts of substances that could create the same symptoms in healthy people.

Hahnemann discovered some of his substances were too strong, often making people sicker, so he started to dilute them even more. At a certain point the dilutions became too weak to work. Now here comes the part that puzzles chemists, doctors and skeptics who think only in a materialistic way.

He decided to try succussion (a term used for rigorous pounding of the bottle) in between dilutions. Amazingly, something happened! The remedies started to work. Somehow Hahnemann got this idea of what we call "potentization" today. We think it may have come from Paracelsus who called something similar "dynamization. No one knows for sure. Some physicists today are working on what actually does happen in the process of succussion.[3] I leave that to the physicists. Being a clinician and a pragmatist, my interest is in clinical results! The bottom line for me is--do people get better or not?

What happened was so surprising, that at one point Hahnemann actually stopped his work because he could not believe the factual results he was getting! At first he noted the effects of his dilutions and succussions were amazing. He started getting real cures. The astounding thing was that the more he diluted and succussed the substance, the stronger the effect it had on the body/mind (the "Vital Force" as we call it now) of the patient. He would dilute it 1:99 parts water (now called the "c" potencies for the word "centesimal"), or 1:9 parts water (now called the "x" potencies for the decimal system--the Latin roman numeral 10); each time he diluted it, he would then succuss it. Each cycle of dilution and succussion was counted as one increased potency, so it went 1c, 2c, 3c etc.

Eventually, after doing this process 12 different times at 1:99 dilution, he knew he had surpassed Avrogadro's number. What THAT means is there was not one molecule of the original substance left in the bottle! Let me say that again, because this point is very important!

> *NOT ONE molecule was left of the original substance, but it worked anyway!*

What does that mean? People were being cured with water that had nothing of the original, material substance in it! It means that the *frequency or energy* of the substance was being received and responded to by the Energetic Matrix (as I like to call the *totality* of the body/mind/energetic field). The term we use in homeopathy, the "Vital Force," is the intelligent force within the body. The results of his treatments led to dramatic changes in the body and the emotions! In fact, as a part of the healing, the whole *frequency* of the person changed--at least we would say that now.

Hahnemann, and the Mystery of Homeopathy

Well, back to Dr. Hahnemann. He was shocked to discover the power of the remedy once it went beyond Avogadro's number (a 12c). He was in as much disbelief as the AMA and all those "quack busters" are today. The difference was, he was a real scientist who couldn't ignore the facts in front of him; the nagging proof of the cures hounded him. He lost his students, and the colleagues who had rallied to his side to learn this new method of cure; but they could not accept that a succussed remedy could cure when there was nothing physical in there. Eventually he had to go back and research more. He discovered that he could continue to succuss and dilute the substance many times over *with stronger and stronger effects on the patient*. Today, you can walk into a health food store and find a remedy in a 30c, which is made by diluting and succussing the substance 30 separate times! Later, many trained in classical homeopathy used even much "higher" potencies, i.e. those shaken and diluted 200 times, 1,000 times, or more! Today it is very common. I know it boggles the mind: that's why so many people are skeptical about homeopathy.

Even today after 30 years of experience, when I make a remedy myself, diluting it and succussing it many times over, it still seems like a very well-washed bottle! My own materialistic mind cannot fathom it, just as it cannot literally fathom that we are all only energy. We are particles alternating with waves, and not the "solid" bodies we think we are. What makes the difference to my materialistic mind is that I know it works, having experienced it personally, and having seen many miracles with it.

I have been fortunate to work in a few holistic medical centers. Arizona has created a license for "Homeopathic Medical Assistant" to doctors who have a homeopathic license for alternative medicine. We work together and help people who either do not choose drugs, cannot tolerate them, or are getting little or no relief from them. Some even continue with their prescription medications for certain conditions, but choose homeopathy to transition into a more natural approach for their overall health and wellbeing. We get good results with homeopathy for injury, common acute illnesses, and chronic mental and physical conditions ...otherwise, I wouldn't be doing this. In Arizona, I am now also called an "HH," a Hahnamannian Healer.

The Self-Regulating Principle: How We, and the Universe, Survive In Every Instant

We are a part of a Self-Regulating Universe: our personal, self-regulating mechanism accounts for our everyday health and the instantaneous results seen with Homeopathy

Our bodies, just like the earth and everything in our Universe, strive for a dynamic form of homeostasis, otherwise called "homeodynamics," by constantly making small or large adjust–ments to maintain a healthy balance. On the earth, small changes are too numerous to be noticed, but a big change can be seen in natural events such as an earthquake or a volcano.

Every day we are exposed to bacteria, viruses, changes in temperature, unhealthy food, pollution, electromagnetic bombardment, and stressors that affect our Energetic Matrix. This Energetic Matrix, which includes our physical body, the energetic fields within us, and our electromagnetic fields surrounding us, is always self-regulating and -correcting to adapt to what otherwise could become a dangerous situation. We live our lives oblivious to the constant fine inner adjustments that make survival possible. It is only when those fine adjustments are not enough to maintain the balance that a bigger change occurs and we get "sick," or an organ gives way, or we die.

Remember, the response to a frequency is no different than a response to an obvious external stressor like smoke or any other toxin. Today our Energetic Matrix is very busy trying to maintain some degree of balance. Think of all the energetic pollution like cell phones and cell towers, electricity, ELF's (extremely low frequency waves), WiFi, radio, TV and microwaves to name only a few obvious ones. If all of these frequencies were audible it would drive us crazy!

A Personal Experience: The Responsive Speed of the Energetic Matrix to Life and Death Conditions

Since homeopathic remedies are frequencies, too, they impinge on us in the same way. A correctly-matching remedy is specifically targeted to what is going on with you. Amazingly, the Energetic Matrix can respond with lightning speed, and specifically does so when perfectly matched with the right remedy (energetic information). See the interview with Bruce Lipton and Karma Singh explaining why this happens. Dr. Lipton speaks of the fact that a chemical reaction (of a pill, for example) uses up 98% of the energy just in the process of released heat required in its chemical reaction. However 100% of the messaging signal is instantly carried to the cells from an energetic signal.
http://www.youtube.com/user/karmahealer#p/a/u/0/WSEKby4 zdok

One of the most dramatic examples I have seen (and there have been too many to mention) was with my former husband. He has a condition known as Marfan's Syndrome, a genetic condition known to cause degeneration of the connective tissue. Abraham Lincoln had it, as do many basketball players. The condition also includes long tubular bones, which create very tall people. When the connective tissues breaks down, it can involve the heart valves, the aorta, and the joints--to name only a few areas where connective tissue is present.

We always knew something could happen to my husband at any time. One afternoon he collapsed at my feet. He rolled around on the floor trying to catch his breath. Before even calling 911, I ran and got three remedies. Because I'd worked with homeopathy in India, I had the opportunity to see its power in many different types of emergencies. Although I had no idea about what was happening inside of him, I knew if I called 911 first, they might arrive before I found the right remedy. The first two remedies I grabbed were for valvular heart problems, which I knew was a possibility. I dropped one in his mouth, nothing happened; I waited 30 seconds, maybe less. Then I tossed the second one into his mouth, nothing happened--he was still rolling on the floor. The third one caused him to take a deep breath, relax, and say "You got the right remedy!" I then called 911. I knew it had to be serious based on the remedy that had worked; it is used for certain kinds of heart problems and internal bleeding. This is a perfect example of how the body is able to instantly self-regulate as a response to the remedy.

I repeated the remedy as needed until they could get him to surgery. The remedies work energetically, being absorbed under the tongue, needing no digestion (Nitroglycerine, a drug used in western medicine for angina, works instantly under the tongue, too). He was subsequently flown to a Phoenix hospital. When I met with the doctor, he told me the inner lining of the aorta had split from his heart to his kidney. We waited for the team to be assembled to replace his aorta with a Dacron shield in an emergency open-heart surgery. The main surgeon, Dr. Dietrich, took me aside and said "You're both extremely lucky. With the extent of the trauma sustained to his body and aorta, very few would have even survived the trip to the hospital. People usually bleed to death internally as the outer aortic wall almost always ruptures soon after the initial dissection (separation)."

I knew from the dramatic shift in seconds after the third remedy, that it had saved his life until he could get the surgery he needed. This could not be called placebo or it would have happened with the first, or even the second remedy we tried. He went into the five-hour surgery twelve hours later; they were able to wait for the full surgical team (after their full day of scheduled surgery) because he was so well-stabilized. The remedy had bought us the time we needed. I watched helplessly as he was wheeled into that life-or-death surgery, knowing I might never see him again. It was a moment I would never want to relive. We were so fortunate to have one of the best cardiac surgeons in the country perform the operation--one who operated only two weeks out of every month!

Afterwards, I supported my husband's recovery with homeopathic Arnica 10M (that means 10,000 dilutions and succussions!) and other remedies that prevented internal bleeding and addressed the trauma from surgery. After open-heart surgeries, everyone has drainage tubes for the internal bleeding. The nurses were confounded as to why there was no drainage at all. Years later, his sister needed the same surgery as a preventative measure, and by using Arnica she had no drainage either.

My First Lesson with an Acute Illness:
More on Self-Regulation!

This is another example of the amazing speed at which our Energetic Matrix can self-correct or rebalance itself. I share these stories because they are so vivid for me, and hopefully will be for you, too. Because I had experienced such relief from my emotions and accompanying chronic symptoms, I was able to accept that homeopathy could handle those well. However, in the very early stages of my study, I still was not so sure about its use for acute illnesses. I remember telling a friend that homeopathy or not, if I ever got another urinary tract infection, I would absolutely go for the antibiotics. After all, I would want those little bacteria to be killed dead. Right? Well, I don't know about you, but I don't offer dares to the "Universe" anymore!

One Friday night I developed a bladder infection. It was excruciatingly painful and I was bleeding. If you've ever had one of these nasty infections, you know what I am talking about. Every time you go to the bathroom (and they say to drink lots of water so you are always running) you think you will die from the cutting, burning pain, which instantly brings tears to your eyes. The alternatives were to go to the emergency room (I didn't have much money and I knew that would be a hefty bill), or wait until morning when the free clinic opened. I would have had to endure severe pain all night and the possibility of a worsening of the symptoms, which I couldn't even imagine! On the other hand, since George Graff was away, my other option was to call my friend Anne who was also studying homeopathy. After a few moments of deliberation, I decided to call Anne.

Anne asked me questions about my symptoms of pain and bleeding, but those would not have been enough to guide her to the right remedy--she needed to know my emotional state. Earlier that day a close friend told me he had to move away from Boulder. I told her I was suddenly feeling really empty and alone again at the thought of his leaving. That was the information she needed. She suggested a remedy in a 1,000c. Of course I took it, still somewhat doubtful but desperate. Within one hour all of my physical symptoms were gone. But the interesting thing was my distress and anxiety over my friend's leaving me melted away! The remedy had triggered a self-regulating response. I started to feel relaxed and "whole" again, almost immediately, even before the pain went completely away. Those who have ever had a bladder infection know it doesn't ever vanish instantly like that. Not even with antibiotics. Don't try this yourself, unless you are under the care of a competent, experienced homeopath. As in all cases, you should consult your healthcare practitioner.

Although many homeopaths would argue with me, if need be, you can take both a remedy and an antibiotic at the same time to start...just know, with the right remedy and potency, you should experience a shift in acute symptoms immediately--often first emotionally, and then physically. That is how you can tell what is working. The antibiotic takes much longer. If the remedy clearly works, well then it is your choice whether to continue with the antibiotic. In my case, the infection didn't come back. Lower potencies will often require a few repetitions to complete the job. Check with your homeopathic practitioner with any questions.

For a complete healing, your Energetic Matrix must rebalance the emotions that are an integral part of your total symptom picture. Your body can't heal if your emotions are in turmoil!

The remedy took me "out of the zone" that included susceptibility to the emotional pain and the bacteria. It is a wild, different concept but perhaps you can get the gist of it. If I had taken an antibiotic, it wouldn't have worked that fast--but most of all, at its best, it would have cleared the infection; but I would have still continued to feel deep emotional fear and pain over the departure of my friend. Those continuing emotions may well have either brought the infection back (recurrent bladder infections are common), or created another "disease" imbalance in my body. This time I was healed from the inside out!

Even after my pain disappeared, my skepticism continued and I needed to prove to myself that I had totally healed. The next morning I decided to go to the clinic to see if my infection had *really* gone away. After all, I thought, maybe it just moved up to my kidneys. That whole experience had never happened to me in the past--a severe bladder infection (which I had had before) disappearing in an hour? It seemed impossible! Where could the infection have gone without antibiotics to kill the bacteria? At the clinic they did a simple test and determined there was no trace of infection. Again, I was astounded. This stuff really did work on bacteria and viruses! No--in fact I have to say it actually doesn't work on the bacteria: it works on the whole person, not the disease! What a concept! Perhaps we could say that it changed the frequency of my whole body so I was no longer a "good host" to the bacteria, or even to fear and emotional pain. I felt stronger, inside and out.

Who Has Used Homeopathy?

In *The Homeopathic Revolution: Why Famous People and Cultural Heroes Choose Homeopathy*, authors Dana Ullman MPH and Peter Fisher MD write about 11 U.S. presidents, seven popes, the British Royal Family, Charles Darwin, David Beckham, Tina Turner, and Mother Teresa--all of whom either advocated for or were benefited by homeopathic treatment. Others include musicians like Ludwig van Beethoven, Robert Schumann, F. Chopin, Sir Yehudi Menuhin, Cher, Paul McCartney, George Harrison, Pete Townshend, Annie Lennox, Bob Weir, Paul Rodgers, Axl Rose, Moby, Jon Faddis, and Dizzy Gillespie.[4] Homeopathy is not a "flakey" thing, but is real and has been proven many times over, here and internationally. It is very well-respected in many countries including India where the severity of many of their diseases requires medicines that work. It is approved there, and in many other countries, by their governments.

During the 1800s, Dr. Fewster Robert Horner (a former President of the British Medical Association) set out to write a paper discrediting homeopathy. According to the research done by Sue Young, presented on the Internet, "Horner was a virulent skeptic of homeopathy who voted against it in the infamous Brighton resolutions of 1851, and who was *solely responsible for suppressing the statistics presented by the London Homeopathic Hospital during the cholera epidemic of 1854. The statistics showed a 66% cure rate with homeopathy vs. a 66% death rate without homeopathy.*" Unconscionable acts like this misrepresentation still happen on occasion today. To his credit, he later became a homeopathic convert and a staunch supporter of homeopathy. He wrote a book, *Homeopathy: Reasons for*

Adopting the Rational System of Medicine, printed in 1860. Horner writes: "Yet up to the very time of instituting my enquiry--it is with humility I make the confession--I was blinded by prejudice and ignorance, like most of the profession in Hull".[5]

Skepticism

Because each person is unique and requires their own remedy (for example, ten Hepatitis patients would require ten totally different remedies), we treat people and their energetic imbalances, not a "named disease." For that reason it is not possible to assess homeopathy very well with double blind studies used in western medicine where it's "a one size fits all" approach, and only one medicine is tested for the "same disease." Actually, interestingly, in reading about quantum physics you discover that there is no such thing as a real, impartial, double blind study because the observer always influences the observed, whether double, or triple blind.

Thanks to Greek homeopath George Vithoulkas, a homeopathic renaissance began again in 1980 in the United States, in spite of the struggle with doubt, skepticism and prejudice, which continues to this day. Strangely, acupuncture has been relatively accepted, but not homeopathy, which at its core is diametrically opposed to western medicine. Almost every American doctor will tell you the results are only because of the placebo effect, because the remedies are only made up of "water." These critics go on and on about how there is nothing left of the original substance; they are right! But they have missed the whole point! First, succussion is required; second, in mainstream medicine, chemistry and biology, thought is materialistic and does not address Energy and the body's own healing response. The truth is although our whole world is only energy and frequency, this concept is ignored; that is why these critics are missing the point. But if they really studied the history of homeopathy, and quantum physics, they would end up doing exactly what Dr. Horner did in the 1800s--recant their position.

Just recently, Dr. Luc Montagnier, the French virologist who won the Nobel Prize in 2008 for discovering the AIDS virus, has surprised the scientific community with his strong support for homeopathic medicine.

See: http://www.huffingtonpost.com/dana-ullman/luc-montagnier-homeopathy-taken-seriously_b_814619.html,

http://www.huffingtonpost.com/dana-ullman/luc-montagnier-homeopathy-taken-seriously_b_814619.html.

Chapter 3

The "Provings": How We Know What the Remedies Create, and Therefore Cure

Important Information for You: How Not to Get in Trouble

Homeopathy: Homeo means "like" and pathos means "suffering in Greek. People ask "how can we know what a remedy will create and therefore cure?" We have what we call "provings." We solicit volunteers, often from homeopaths themselves, or students in homeopathic schools, and give them an unnamed remedy to take a number of times. New symptoms are recorded daily, sometimes even hourly, on all levels--mental, emotional and physical. A supervisor calls daily to monitor all changes. Then symptoms are collected and studied. Patterns are noted. From this information, a total "symptom picture" is compiled. Based on the substance's effects, we can predict what combination of symptoms the remedy may cure. I emphasize *combination*, because classical homeopaths never give a remedy based on one symptom; it is the combination of symptoms on the physical, mental and emotional levels that bring us to the correct remedy for the whole person.

In reading information from the homeopaths who had done provings on themselves in the past, I remember thinking these were the "saints" or "martyrs" of homeopathy. They often pushed the proving far more than we would today. Years ago, I read the report of one such doctor who wrote, "I felt very sick, and got up and vomited a coffee ground substance, and then I took another dose." In my mind I thought, *You did what?* These people were dedicated enough to really want to understand the illness pattern in the extreme and see what the remedy would create, and therefore cure.

Overdoing Any Remedy, or Having an "Aggravation"

It is important to know that you can also overdo any remedy, in other words create your own proving. This happens if you take a remedy when you don't, or no longer, need it. Should that happen, stop taking the remedy and wait for symptoms indicators to calm down. Often, at the end of the reaction, there may be a clearing of those symptoms.

As in any use of a potentized remedy, in rare cases, an aggravation is possible with a HeartFusion™ remedy. That means the symptoms may get worse before they get better. So far in my work, I have only seen this three times in over 135 people with my HeartFusion™ method which incorporates homeopathic principles. What happened in those three people was that on taking the HeartFusion™, their emotions or physical sensations increased in intensity. Should this happen to you with the HeartFusion™ method, there are two options. The easiest is to spray it again; this may move the energy sufficiently for you to quickly feel better. The other option is to make it stronger and take it immediately again. On one rare occasion, we took it up to a 30 potency--and then the magic instantly happened! The instantaneous shift was dramatic! The only time it was advisable to stop a HeartFusion™ was when one woman got enthusiastic and sprayed it 20 or more times in one day! With more traditional homeopathic remedies, my advice is to stop the remedy right away if symptoms flare up.

Suppression and Hering's Laws of Cure: Are You Healed or Just Suppressed?

The following information may be more than some of you ever wanted to know about homeopathy. There are some important points I'd like to share, especially about suppression, so bear with me for this part even if you are considering jumping ahead.

In homeopathy, we believe the Vital Force is an intelligent, interactive Being; it is not passive, waiting to be forced to comply with what we believe it should do. In western medicine, the "voice" of your Vital Force or your Energetic Matrix is constantly being suppressed by drugs. That "voice" is another word for your "symptoms." For example, if you ate something bad, the Vital Force might create nausea, vomiting, diarrhea or all of the above, to cleanse the system of the poison. If these symptoms were to be suppressed, the poisons would remain in the body. The correct homeopathic remedy will stimulate the Vital Force to rebalance itself and take you out of the "zone" of susceptibility to the poison or virus or bacteria. Recovery from food poisoning or fever or virus is then amazingly fast, without suppression. It amazes me-after all these years! I have witnessed this again and again in India, here, and in other countries.

The Effects of Suppressing Emotions

The same principle relating to suppression applies to deep emotions. If natural responses and emotions are allowed to run their course, health can be regained. Let's use the example of grief. Many doctors immediately prescribe anti-depressants when a patient has a good reason to grieve--like a death in the family or a disease. Instead of encouraging the normal grieving process to run its course, we, as healers, want to make everyone happy and comfortable. Our society allows no room for this either--no one is paid leave to process their traumas. Drugs flat line emotions so people cannot process emotions naturally, nor can they experience the wonderful "highs" of life. The young, now being drugged by the millions with anti-depressants and Ritalin, never learn how to deal with their real-life emotions.

Suppression of emotional or physical symptoms can cause serious mental and physical repercussions. Some would call this the "male model of healing": "Stomp out those bad symptoms and get on with your life!" However, the "feminine model" fits in better with homeopathy--gently remind the Energetic Matrix it has work to do and let it naturally respond! Why is the U.S. so far behind many of the other countries for good health when we spend more on medical care than anyone else? One answer is because there is so much suppression here.

Sooner or later, after a suppression, our Energetic Matrix finds a way to continue its expression of the original imbalance since it was never addressed or allowed to self-correct. This is done either by side-stepping the drug and re-expressing the same symptoms, or by expressing the imbalance on an even deeper level. In homeopathy, in general, we usually consider the mental/emotional level to be deeper than the physical one. If we are deeply emotionally or mentally imbalanced, even suicidal, the limitation to our life may be greater than if we had a less limiting physical symptom. Of course, this schemata gets much more complicated. For a more in-depth discussion of this see George Vithoulkas' book.[6] In the new technology I am about to present, it is important to remember we are not suppressing emotions, but facing them head on homeopathically, in order to stimulate your own self-corrective mechanism.

Homeopathy's Philosophy and "Laws of Cure" as Discovered by Constantine Hering

For example, if you are depressed and have a skin condition, your depression HAS TO improve first, or at least simultaneously. If your skin gets better but you become depressed, nobody did you any favors! You may get referred to a psychiatrist for your new depression, but he/she will never understand that your depression may have begun, or been aggravated, due to use of a suppressive cream on your skin (like Cortisone). Doctors are not trained to look at the whole person from that perspective, nor do they know how to interpret the changing symptoms. Classically-trained homeopathic practitioners do just that; they look at the whole person. For a more detailed explanation of the "Laws of Cure" which apply to all healing modalities, even western medicine, go to Appendix 1 in the back of the book.

Remember, as with all healing modalities, there can be suppression with homeopathy *if* the remedy chosen does not address the whole symptom constellation, including the deep underlying emotional issues. This is a very important piece to keep in mind. If these issues are not addressed, sooner or later worse symptoms, seemingly unrelated, may ultimately manifest.

Consider the challenging emotions in *your* life; these are critical to the HeartFusion™ process.

Chapter 4

Addressing Our Emotions: Do We Focus on the Positive or Work on Our "Shadow" Side?

There is a philosophy in New Age thinking that says focus on the positive and ignore the "negative" emotions like fear, hurt or anger. By always creating positive visualizations or affirmations rather than the "negative ones" it is said that you will attract and create the wonderful reality you always wanted. Witness the famous DVD "The Secret." There is a hope and an assumption that the negative part will just melt away when we focus only on the positive. We wonder "Can't we just ignore our stuff and go onto something more pleasant?" Wouldn't that be nice? I would love that! Sometimes changing the energy in a particular situation will work miracles; however, ultimately the old issues just keep coming back over and over in one form or another (like suppressed symptoms). These deep issues take more than positive thinking and feeling to be transformed. Psychologists and therapists take issue with this "positive only" approach, claiming the need for deep understanding of these issues is necessary. So, who is right?

Social and Psychological Ramifications of Suppression

Let's look at the suppression of emotions for a moment. Suppression can keep us dishonest in our relationships with ourselves and with others. I remember when the whole EST craze was happening in the 80s. I knew people who were facing financial ruin, and when you asked them how they were, they would put on a smile and say enthusiastically "fine!" What kind of relationship can you have with someone who will not speak the truth about what they are really feeling? I know a number of "New Agers" who are like that now. It is also true that someone who constantly complains is a turn off, but so is "faked" joy.

Suppression of feelings also requires a huge amount of energy, since you are holding down whatever is not being expressed. In addition, this means that you cannot receive the "Light" or the joy that would otherwise be available to you. When you think of someone with a "stiff upper lip," you don't see a person who is vibrant and fun-loving, spreading joy in their wake! This constant suppression creates energy blockages that cause "dis-ease," very much like a physical toxin! Expressions like "It is eating me up" and "It makes me sick" reflect back this reality. How can the self-regulating or self-corrective principle come into play when we are holding ourselves in so tightly that nothing can move or flow? Eventually, the Energetic Matrix gives up and says, "OK, this is what you want? This is what I will do. I will not move, change, or heal myself. I will surrender to what you want: this stasis of imbalance. I will put all of my energy into keeping the status quo of suppression."

These rigid places have to be freed for our total Being (our Energetic Matrix) to be able to breathe, expand, and evolve! Then more of our energy, light and love can shine through and help to connect us with that ultimate positive "field" of Love and joy which exists behind all thought. Believe it or not, it's always there, just not always accessible to our conscious awareness. The more we suppress, however, the deeper these patterns and rigidities go. Just like suppressed physical symptoms, these suppressed emotions show up deep inside the body. So you see why we cannot pretend our pain is gone when it is not. The body never lies. At a certain point, something has to give; it could be our physical body, or even our sanity. Then what? In our society we turn to drugs and suppress our symptoms even more.

Patterns of Pain

Some believe we are here on this planet to grow. If that is true, then it is no surprise that life will present challenges that are not only uncomfortable, but sometimes even extremely painful. Teething is painful for a baby, but it is also necessary part of development. Therein lies the problem: these "patterns" or imprints of our pain are cumulative; they create a "lens" through which we view our life experiences. They have created deep "grooves" in our Energetic Matrix; in fact we may have even been born with some of them. Some say these patterns are in our DNA. Others say they are due to the chemicals held in our mother's womb reflecting her emotional states. It doesn't matter. The fact is, we are born with physical and emotional imbalances. Then along comes life, with its challenges and difficulties, and we are affected. We respond in certain ways as the previous memories, or patterns, attach to these new experiences, and these create the corresponding neuropathways in our brains.

Back to Creating Positive Thought:
Is that the Answer?

There have been some amazing suggestions and research around how we create our reality with our thoughts, thereby creating a field of energy in and around us (i.e. our whole Energetic Matrix) that gives rise to more of the same. So, in that genre of thinking and literature, we have been guided to go into the "field of positive thought" to attract what we want. We have also learned that words and thought are not enough; we must create the emotional energy that accompanies those thoughts to truly activate that field of creation.

This information is very powerful, yet many of you, like me, may have had times when it felt like we were on something akin to a "moving sidewalk" at the airport. "Life" seized us and pulled us in a direction we could not seem to stop or change. Events leading up to a major tragedy, or a divorce, or a dramatic shift in our lives may often feel like that. You may have seen it coming, but no amount of swimming against the tide of life, or positive thinking to create "good energies" or a different outcome, could have changed the flow. Often later, in retrospect, we realize it was the best thing that ever happened to us. But at the time it would have felt like the end of the world; if we knew how, we would have stopped the flow and stayed with the familiar. As a typical example, many people have experienced their life opening and transforming positively after, or maybe because of, a divorce, or a loss of a job, or an illness. However, at those times, initially the pain of change may feel unbearable and, like nausea, there seems to be no way to escape it. It may take a long time before we have the perspective that allows us to say: "It was the best thing that ever happened to me!"

I am always put off when someone says, in a very glib way, "Just get out of that space! Think positively! Get over it!" I have often thought if you told that same glib person their mother just died, or their spouse, or their child, see how fast they "get over it!" In the process of life we get knocked around, and often we get stuck in an emotion for a much longer time than we would like...for some, even for a lifetime. We have all met bitter, angry, or grieving individuals who continue to be crippled by their emotions all their lives. The question arises, "What tools can we utilize to help us move out of these difficult emotions that seem to stick to us and often reverberate like a theme throughout our lives?" Is it enough to simply focus on "positive thoughts" to enter the "Love Field"? At difficult, painful times is it even possible? I remember my experience living in the spiritual community. It was wonderful and incredible; I spent a lot of time in meditation and in bliss. I had never known such ecstasy and I was given many tools to enter that "Field:" both in my daily life, and in meditation. When our "stuff" would come up, our instructions were to return to our heart center and to focus on love. I did that for years. Yet my reactions to situations in life would come along to pull me out of that joy. Those "negative" imprinted patterns in my psyche never quite went away! Sound familiar? We all experience that in our own ways. I discovered that even with the years of meditation I had done before, during and after living in the community, trying to focus only on love could be helpful, but it wasn't the "whole enchilada." In fact, sometimes it wasn't even possible!

Homeopathy has shown itself to be a powerful tool for change. Practitioners and patients have seen that it is real and that it works. The big question is "How can we *all* break these patterns that are so deeply ingrained in our brains, our chemistry, and our Energetic Matrix; what can we do for ourselves?"

Applying the principle of "like cures like" in a unique way may provide a powerful key to our process of deep transformation.

The HeartFusion™ Method Can Take You Home!

- *What if someone gave you a tool that not only lessened the pain, but put you into a place of balance, and left you feeling like you had come home to yourself?*

- *What if that tool were something you could do on your own in your home?*

- *What if that tool had many other implications, limited only by your imagination?*

- *What if that tool allowed you to access that place of release, of peace and a sense of wellbeing? Even if you felt far from it?*

- *How would that impact your life? Your family? Other relationships?*

- *Would you want that tool?*

- *More importantly, would you remember to use it?*

While we may need and want to be consciously in and aware of that "Ultimate Field" of peace, consciousness and love, we also need the tools to really get there, tools that dissolve the old patterns that keep pulling us back to our old thoughts and ways. If not used correctly, even visualization and imagination can become a suppression. You cannot cheat or fool "life"--which is really YOURSELF; you can try to pretend that everything is great--but if it is not, sooner or later something has to give!

The HeartFusion™ method is powerful in the process of transformation and healing. "Life" seems to bring us the same patterns over and over again in a very homeopathic way; it is confronting us and giving us the opportunity to respond and grow (self-regulate), much like in the profound movie "Groundhog Day." It would be wonderful if we could support ourselves to move on in a less painful way. This is what I want to address with our new method: how do we really get there without having to struggle so much? I am not saying this is the only way, but I am saying this method has worked for just about everyone in my workshops and my clients. It can also be combined with almost any other modality if you so desire.

"Cosmic Homeopathy?"

Looking at our planet, it is easy to see the mess we are in: extreme pollution, corruption, violence and greed. Then we look at how the planet is reflecting back to us: mega earthquakes, storms, typhoons, tornadoes, droughts and floods. One can only wonder: are we not being asked to change our ways? In almost an allegorical way, are we not being challenged to move from greed, corruption and competition into cooperation and love? Could this be the planet's ultimate homeopathic prescription to humanity for the necessary growth and transformation of our species and the saving of our planet?

Nourishing Ourselves

I believe it is vitally important to find ways to feed and access the love that lays deep within us, whatever the form. For some it may be communing with nature, for others praying or meditating, or connecting with "The Divine," or "God," or our own perception of our "Higher Power." If you are not familiar with meditation, which is a powerful method to quiet the mind and open the heart, please see the Appendix 3 at the end of this book. Some will immediately think-"I can't do that!" But in fact there are many ways to "trick" the mind to quiet itself, so you can feel your true essence--who you really are behind the chatter of the mind.

Chapter 5

Finding the Right Remedy: The Science and Challenge of Homeopathy and Homeopathic Imponderabelia

There have been a few times in my life when I went through a "Dark Night of the Soul." As I described earlier, sometimes homeopathy worked miraculously, literally saving my life; but I must say there were other times when finding the right remedy was challenging. There are a few thousand remedies available (some more researched than others) with new ones being researched every day. Homeopathy is very scientific in its provings, principles, and Laws of Cure; but it is very much of an art to find the right remedy (not so unlike western medicine when different drugs are tried until one has a positive effect without many side effects). The practitioner must be very skilled, and still sometimes finding the right remedy can be a challenge. Sophisticated software has been developed, with over one million symptoms listed and all the remedies known to cure each one. There are programs with word searching capabilities in over 650 books and old journals, and other programs designed to help the trained practitioner to ask the right questions to find the right remedy. Still, it is a challenge for the best of homeopaths to match the perfect remedy to their client every time.

A Note of Caution

In an attempt to make the miracles of homeopathy more accessible to the untrained homeopath (most medical doctors and other health care professionals who have not studied homeopathy in depth), computerized devices were designed. These devices are supposed to be programmed to find the remedy quickly so the operator doesn't need to be educated in the complexities of homeopathy. But impressive as they look, I have seen dangerous prescribing by those who were uneducated about the depths of homeopathy. Any modality powerful enough to heal is also powerful enough to cause imbalance; from drugs to homeopathic remedies, herbs, and even to acupuncture! Although their developers may have good intentions, they are mostly uneducated in the subtleties of homeopathy. Computerized programs may prescribe many remedies and potencies at once. This can be confusing to the Energetic Matrix.

Similarly there are companies that market mixtures of different (often dangerously high-potency) remedies, which they pitch to homeopathically uneducated healthcare professionals as a quick fix. These combinations can cause problems. Homeopathically untrained practitioners don't understand (regardless of their licenses) nor do untrained practitioners know what warning signs to look for, like provings, suppressions, and disruptions. Finding the perfect, matching remedy (called the constitutional remedy) for each person is ideal, but still doesn't always happen. In addition, there are more people needing help than there are well-trained practitioners. It can take years to become really good. In fact, practitioners share new information at seminars and conferences all the time; it is a lifetime pursuit.

With the new system of HeartFusion™ I present here, everyone can benefit from healing based on homeopathic principles. Times are changing--we don't know what external support for mental and physical ills may be available in the future, or for those who cannot afford drugs or treatment. For example, people in areas of natural disasters do not always have access to drugs, herbs or even remedies; but HeartFusion™ is a technique that could help anyone as long as there is water and a container.

Children and Homeopathy

Homeopathy has always been amazing for babies and children of all ages. I have seen many homeopathic miracles--whether the issues seem mostly physical (like recurring ear or bronchial infections), or mental--like "ADD" or "ADHD," or any of the other "syndromes" that now have been given insurance codes. I have watched children with deep fears, nightmares, or a strong "mean streak" be transformed into balanced, happy children. Of course, there are other variables like parenting, etc. But in any case, the child will be positively supported with the right remedy. Catch a child who is already veering off balance, treat them homeopathically, and you have changed a life forever! I have seen children go from being the most difficult to the most delightful literally overnight. The results with homeopathy can be that profound.

You can only imagine how frustrating it is to have this knowledge and be in a country where homeopathy is ridiculed, unappreciated and unknown! At first, when I would read about a child that had been traumatized by kidnapping or some other terrible occurrence in their lives, and I would have to restrain myself from contacting the parents to tell them about homeopathy for trauma and shock! They would have never believed me! I have had the opportunity to treat children who had such traumas.

One child had been witness to an intruder coming into the home and tying his parents up while they looted the house. The child had managed to hide but was totally traumatized, and had many symptoms as a result. A single dose of a high potency remedy for fear and trauma (in this case, Aconite) ended his nightmares and anxiety. Seeing children transform like that after a remedy has been worth all the years and money I have spent on my education!

And Another Leap…Imponderabilia

This next leap is a critical one for you to understand in the HeartFusion™ process. Most of our remedies come from the plant, mineral and animal kingdoms.

Another kind of remedy that we have in homeopathy is called an "imponderabelia." Remedies called "imponderabelia" are made from pure energies, rather than physical substances. Examples include electricity, x-ray, radiation, North Pole, South Pole, total magnet, the sun's rays, the moon's rays, and others. Water is exposed to the specific energetic, like x-raying it, or placing it out in the sunlight. Then it is treated like any other remedy: the water is potentized through succussion and dilution.

The first time that I ever used such a remedy was Electricitas 1M (1M stands for 1,000 cycles of dilution and succussion) or homeopathic electricity. That was 24 years ago. I had a client who was referred by a doctor who couldn't figure out what to do with her. She had a history of many shock treatments in her youth. Those resulted in many strange symptoms that severely limited her. They were not just emotional symptoms, but physical symptoms as well, including severe diarrhea immediately after eating. She could never share a meal with any friends or go to a restaurant for fear of how she would react physically. I went to Dr. John Henry Clark's three-volume "Dictionary of the Materia Medica" and looked up homeopathic electricity known as "Electricitas." There were pages of information about homeopathic electricity and what the proving had created in healthy subjects; however, many of her symptoms were not even listed. Nevertheless, given her history of the brutal shock treatments from her early 20s, and the fact the symptoms had continued for another 20 years, I decided to try it. It was early on for me in homeopathy; I only had about six years of experience, and I was a little unsure about whether this "imponderabelia" remedy would work or not, but I I decided to try it.

After taking the remedy, she reported immediately feeling a shift in her energy; her heart started beating fast, her body flushed for a few minutes, and then she felt a deep sense of release. Slowly over the next week her symptoms started to melt away. Over the course of a few weeks, all of the severe symptoms that had limited her life had disappeared. I myself was amazed that water, with electricity passed through it, shaken and diluted 1,000 different times, actually could have any effect at all!

New Medical Proof of Imponderabelia: The Imprinting of Water in the UK

I was excited to read that in the UK a hospital conducted an experiment to see if certain patients with electrical sensitivities would respond to a remedy made from frequencies of electrical devices. A frequency from the electronics in question was "imprinted into water, potentized, and used in the same way as allergists use their dilutions." This was done "even though there was no chemical component present," only the electronic imprinting. The original reference relating to Breakspear Hospital, Hemel Hempstead by Rea et al explains that a double-blind trial at the Environmental Health Centre was conducted. Subjects responded with 100% success and 0% response to placebos." I got this information from the following reference, which strangely has since been removed from the Internet: http://www.publications.parliament.uk/pa/cm200910/cmselect/cmsctech/memo/homeopathy/ucm0802.htm. The response to this search was "The requested object does not exist on this server. The link you followed is either outdated, inaccurate, *or the server has been instructed not to let you have it.*" You be the judge as to why it was removed!

Fortunately this information was published in another place too, and so far is still available: http://hpathy.com/homeopathy-scientific-research/homeopathy-%E2%80%93-how-it-works-and-how-it-is-done-2/[7] Scroll past the ads to the study by Cyril W. Smith if you want to see the technical details.

You would think that the research would have stirred great scientific excitement and numerous articles, but as you can see, it did not. Instead it was initially ignored, and now worse, removed. At this time there are attacks on homeopathy in the UK in an attempt to block it from the National Health Service, disregarding its history there, as well as present-day research. Perhaps that is why the study has disappeared....

Everything is Frequency

Everything in our Universe is made up of atoms. Those atoms are all the same except that they have different frequen–cies-- from wood, to metal to people. Our radios, TVs, and cell phones are also receivers and transmitters of frequency, just like we are. Our brains put out frequencies just as they receive them.

This all takes us back to the truth that everything, *everything*, is frequency, and water records frequency. Records from all over the world of homeopathic usage by doctors and laymen have proved that potentization of water encoded with frequency affects everything: body, mind and emotions. Once again, my purpose in writing this book is to share information with you. Some of the "scientific proof" can be researched in my bibliography, as well as the Internet references given in the text. But the real proof can be found in the history of homeopathy, with the cures during epidemics, and from the people and doctors who have seen the results with their own eyes. Ultimately, it will be proved yet again by your own experiences in this new way of creating and using remedies. Funny how you can't prove something to most scientists unless they believe it in the first place! Again, I present this in these steps so that you can understand the concept along the way leading to this new approach.

Chapter 6

Homeopathic Prophylaxis (Prevention) and What Can Be Made into a Remedy? Beyond Vaccination

Making a Disease Remedy for Prevention: Recent Proof From Cuba

There is one very recent paper on the use of homeopathic prophylaxis (in other words, using homeopathic remedies to prevent disease). Homeopathic history abounds with examples, but this one is from three years ago. Cuba is a country like India, and many others, where homeopathy is accepted and used by the government. In Cuba, there is a serious disease, Leptospirosis, which occurs mostly after hurricanes when the sanitation is poor. A few thousand people contract it every year in spite of vaccinations, and there are always some deaths from it. In 2007, 2.5 million people were given homeopathic Leptospirosis 200c once two weeks apart, before the season started, at the nominal cost of $200,000. Only 10 people out of 2.5 million got the disease after receiving the homeopathic remedy! It was the largest experiment ever done that proved homeopathic medicines work. It was done again with similar stunning results the following year in 2008, and presented at an international conference on Homeoprophylaxsis in Havana in 2009.

Originally I found it on this site:
http://www.hpathy.com/papersnew/ruchira-Prevention-Epidemic-Leptospirosis-Cuba.asp

But recently I came up with an "Error" message! So try this one:
http://homeopathyresource.wordpress.com/2009/01/01/successful-use-of-homeopathy-in-over-5-million-people-reported-from-cuba/

and also:
http://www.finlay.sld.cu/nosodes/en/ProgramaNOSODES2008Eng.pdf.

For more information on the history of homeopathic prophylaxis see:
http://homeopathyplus.com.au/category/immunisation/

We are very ethnocentric in the US, i.e. *we only believe what we are told by our own media and our own so-called "experts."* I wanted you to understand this part so you can have a good basis for understanding what is to come. This particular Cuban experiment made use of isopathy--the treatment of the same thing by the same thing, rather than "homeopathy" which is based on using something *similar* to treat the condition. It can work well, and worked for this prevention method!

You yourself can try isopathy for protection when you or your children get sick; you can try to protect others in the family, or even the sick person in question by making a remedy from the disease itself. In some ways this is close to what we will do too, but in a very different way for very different reasons. We will primarily be focusing on the emotions. For more information on making your own disease remedies, see information in Appendix 2.

Some homeopaths will argue saying that the HeartFusion™ method is isopathy and therefore less effective than homeopathy; actually emotions are very mercurial, the "same ones" changing slightly in different situations, so I think the HeartFusion™ method actually is homeopathic.

More on The Principle of Self-Regulation and Correction

The whole Universe, as my magnificent and inspirational friend Dr. Ashok Gangadean pointed out, is self-corrective and self-regulating. If you were to look up those phrases on the Internet, you would see that they apply to everything from descriptions in astrophysics to cardiology and microbiology. We as humans are no exception; neither is the homeopathic process! It doesn't matter that a remedy may be one part per million or one part per billion.

Quantity is not the issue or point of focus. What matters is the response from the Energetic Matrix to that particular energy!

Until western science understands this concept, the scientific community will continue to claim homeopathy to be a hoax. In some medical disciplines, the use of the self-regulatory process is already in use. For example, in certain methods of brain training, the imbalance of the brain's mental patterning is mirrored back to itself in order to stimulate a rebalancing through the self-corrective mechanism. Dr. Sung Lee in Sedona Arizona uses this method.

See http://www.brainwellcenter.com/Scientific.html.

In allopathic (western) medicine there are a few drugs that unwittingly make use of this self-corrective principle--namely Ritalin (a form of speed used for hyperactivity), and Digitalis, otherwise known as Lanoxin, for cardiac fibrillation. Yet, the principle continues to goes unrecognized by those who criticize homeopathy.

We all know the body has the most profound ability to heal itself. Many amazing cures with only pure drinking water have been documented, allowing the body to do its work uninterrupted. When you think about it, headaches, stomach aches, influenza, colds and all sorts of conditions heal by the work of the body alone. The fact that we live through these acute illnesses instead of dying is a testament to our body's ability to heal itself! It is noteworthy that antibiotics are useless against any viral condition, yet without medical intervention we generally recover on our own. However, the Energetic Matrix can work so much faster when stimulated, challenged, and reminded to do its job using homeopathic principles.

Symptoms

The body's self-corrective mechanism is also always working to protect us from the many millions of bacteria, carcinogens and other toxins that bombard our system daily. Like a tightrope walker who teeters to the left and then the right to maintain balance, our body is in a constant state or self-regulation as we obliviously go through our day. Maybe we feel a little more tired one day, or our nose runs, or we get an upset stomach, but that is a part of the work of our Vital Force, bringing us back to a level of a "homeodynamics" or balance. In chronic conditions, I see our Vital Force as being in a static state of accepting the "balanced imbalance" and not being motivated to correct it. Basically, I say "balanced" because you still continue on in life, with physical or emotional pain, or with exhaustion, in one way or another.

This book reaches out beyond the scientific community, to all of you, giving you the power to heal yourself. I have seen and felt the reality of this method and I want YOU to have the benefit of it. This is a self-help revolution, giving you the tools and power to heal and transform yourself. This HeartFusion™ method, which we are building up to, stimulates your Energetic Matrix to naturally self-correct, just like we are meant to. It is the same way the Universe naturally self-corrects on every level, in every moment.

Chapter 7
Water, Frequency, Dr. Masaru Emoto, and Medical Research

Homeopathy and Water

Homeopathic remedies are made in water, and water is much more mysterious than we can imagine. Long ago I heard that water had memory. An example was: if you freeze water at a very high altitude, its crystalline structure would be different from freezing it at sea level; yet if you took that same high-altitude frozen crystal, and defrosted it, then froze it again at sea level, it would carry the memory of the previous high-altitude structure. That was all I knew about the mystery of water, the medium for homeopathy. It explained very little about the homeopathic process, which was to change my life many times over.

The making of a homeopathic remedy incorporates the concept that water has what we would call "memory." A few physicists are only now beginning to unlock these secrets; some say it is related to biophotons[8].

Big Pharma (big pharmaceutical companies) is not interested in pouring lots of money into researching something that cannot be patented, can be made by the educated, and hence be unprofitable. In fact, their commitment is to discredit it. In this country, the drug industry in power and money is second only to the petrochemical industry.

After homeopathy, the next clue in my immense treasure hunt of life was discovered about 15 years ago in an Australian magazine (which, unfortunately, I have since lost). It showed homeopathic remedies frozen, then sliced and viewed under a microscope. Every remedy, and every potency of that remedy, showed a different pattern of brilliant colors! It was similar to Dr. Emoto's work, and quietly preceded it by many years.

Dr. Masaru Emoto and the Water Crystals: How He Changed Our View of Life!

The "coup d'état" was Dr. Emoto's amazing discoveries, revealed in his book *The Hidden Messages in Water*[9]. For those not familiar with him, he is the famous Japanese researcher who visually proved that water is imprinted by frequency/energy from thought, emotion, voice and music. Water is therefore constantly being affected by its environment. He showed, through many interesting experiments, that water changed its frozen crystalline structure, as water itself responded to different frequencies. This was observed after thoughts, emotions or words had been projected onto the water, then the water was frozen and the crystals that formed were photographed. His research shocked, thrilled and amazed me (and much of the world!). You can see the proof in photographs of the resulting frozen crystalline structures at http://www.hadousa.com/photos.html.

Also see these photographs for yourself on YouTube: http://www.youtube.com/watch?v=Ss69kfHqN1A

As Dr. Emoto says (quoted from his web site): "Thus far then we can literally see how the state of water varies greatly even though it is the same H_2O. Geometric order, in hexagonal form, appears in frozen crystals of water exposed to positive influence. And yet negative influence can be so powerful that crystals do not form at all." We see, instead, other patterns appearing in the frozen water, often looking rather ominous.

In his famous initial discovery, Dr. Emoto took lake water that was so polluted that no frozen crystalline structure could be found, and showed the effects on it after prayers of love and gratitude were recited over the lake. The pictures after water had been prayed over showed a beautiful crystalline structure in the ice. Later photographs of frozen water demonstrated the effects of different words, thoughts and sounds. These pictures still astound and delight us as they are shown in his books and on his website. Thanks to Dr. Emoto, we can actually see proof that our thoughts give off vibration (which is literally the frequency coming from our brains and even our hearts and our bodies) that can be seen as measurable patterns in the ice!

In his book *The True Power of Water,* Dr. Emoto[10] speaks of actually talking to water and thanking it, in advance, for creating healing frequencies (he uses the word, "Hado") for diseases and specific people. He then uses that water as a healing medicine for them. We will see that other research confirms the healing power of water. His approach is brilliant. You will explore a similar approach later in the book that is different because we integrate homeopathic principles and methods. It is exciting to see both approaches and how the two

can work for our healing. I am in deep gratitude for his discoveries, which made possible this new HeartFusion™ approach. Although he talks about his system not being strictly scientific, as different crystals may be formed in different moments from the same words (like all of nature--no two things are ever totally alike!) the important piece for our work is that the imprinting of water with thought and words is proven and valid. Some scientists have concluded that water has its own responsive "consciousness." For images of different water crystals from waterways around the world see:
http://www.hadousa.com/places.html

Chapter 8
Vibrations: Medical Research into Frequency

When you think about it, everything that exists is made up of atoms; vibration and frequency gives the collection of atoms form. All aspects of physics, like String Theory and Quantum Mechanics, teach and demonstrate what most forms of regular medicine do not even consider. That is what keeps homeopathy in the realm of disbelief for western scientists. Einstein himself said "The field (i.e. energy) is the sole governing agency of the particle" (i.e. matter).

The general public is mostly unaware that there are devices that can measure the frequencies and energy of every thought (another form of proof that the brain gives off frequencies, just as Emoto's water crystal photography shows that thoughts affect water!). "SQUID" (superconducting quantum interference device) gradiometers and magnetometers are most commonly used in Magnetoencephalography (MEG) to measure the magnetic fields produced by the brain. Scientists can now use those fields of energy to manipulate our external world. Examples include using only brain activity to guide the functioning and manipulation of computers, wheelchairs and even planes, to name a few. There are other means of measuring and even translating patterns of thoughts into discernible emotions and even words. Only a few examples are: the Russians, The Heartmath Institute in the US, Dr. Glen Rein, and independently, Dr. Bruce Lipton. They have discovered that emotions (stemming from a heart-centered place--not just the brain) with words, can effect and change DNA. Dr. Dana Tomasino's paper referred to on the following link called "New Technology Provides Scientific Evidence of Water's Capacity to Store and Amplify Weak Electromagnetic and Subtle Energy Fields."[11] It has also been shown, by Dr. Rein also of the HeartMath Institute, that DNA relaxes and "unwinds" (activates) with positive thought, whereas it shuts down with fear and stress.

Additional Research from Russia

These are some additional pieces of information from Russian science that prove, once again, that the power of the mind and frequency has an effect on our body and the world around us. I find them profound and inspiring. I discovered them on a wonderful website of Dr. John Mallon, physicist, called http://www.thehealinguniverse.com.[12] All the following references can be found and papers downloaded from his amazing online source:
http://www.thehealinguniverse.com/library.html.[13]

This fascinating thought, from Dr. John Mallon's site (see part three of three free online videos): "We are a Universe of frequency and frequency vibrates through moisture or water. Water is the medium that communicates telepathically through our brains."

Please take the time to read slowly and ponder the implications of the following Russian references from Mallon's website that are quickly becoming some of the most quoted research on energy on the Internet.

"Research was done with water in 2 pitchers--instantaneously when changing the frequency of one, the other automatically changes in the same way. We are learning that the thought that changes our body chemistry and even our DNA, is based in water." [14]

Consider the implications of this...

Water is everywhere--in other people and in the air. What are the implications for you and others when you change your thoughts? Thoughts actually affect the moisture in air around you, and even the water in other people's bodies too!

From this perspective, we must ask how we affect each other? How do we affect the environment in a room?

DNA, removed many miles from a biological donor, registers identical and instantaneous responses to changes in the emotional state of the donor."[15]

Perhaps space and time mean less than we ever thought! This reminds us of the studies done on plants, animals and their owners in "The Secret Life of Plants"[16] and more recent research, including the ideas of "entanglement."

Using a programmed laser, "Frog embryos can be transformed to become salamander embryos simply by transmitting salamander embryo DNA information"[17]

Can we begin to imagine the power of frequency? If we can change the very DNA of one species into another, how deeply does frequency affect us? Through that alone, we can begin to fathom the mysteries and power of frequency.

So, if we knew how, we could transmit a frequency to ourselves and thereby change our own DNA, our genetics, our programming and our physical and emotional expressions... all of which are on biochemical *and* energetic levels. The power of frequency is the key for understanding this...and the HeartFusion™ method.

Would this change on all of our levels be so different from turning frogs into salamanders?

"Hypnosis, which is focused suggestion, demonstrates profound effects on DNA."[18]

This has huge implications proving the ability of the mind to change our bodies; but aside from homeopathy, until now we have not had access to the power of a physical and energetic substance to stimulate the desired changes in our brains and DNA. Therefore, our subconscious minds have continued to run with their old programming.

"There is evidence for a whole new type of medicine in which DNA can be influenced and reprogrammed by words and frequencies WITHOUT cutting out and replacing single genes."[19]

"This, too, was experimentally proven! Living DNA substance (in living tissue, not in vitro) will always react to language-modulated laser rays and even to radio waves, if the proper frequencies are being used. This finally and scientifically explains why affirmations, autogenous training, hypnosis and the like can have such strong effects on humans and their bodies. It is entirely normal and natural for our DNA to react to language. While western researchers cut single genes from the DNA strands and insert them elsewhere, the Russians enthusiastically worked on devices that can influence the cellular metabolism through suitable modulated radio and light frequencies and thus repair genetic defects." [20]

What does this tell you about frequencies, thoughts and your own Energetic Matrix?

If words themselves are so powerful, can the *frequency* of words and emotions be used to heal the mental and emotional as well?

"Exposure to recorded DNA-wave information from living seeds, encoded on radio waves, can resuscitate seeds that had been destroyed by radioactivity."

"When a laser hologram, generated from a healthy raspberry plant, is transmitted to a raspberry plant tumor (callus) it causes the callus to develop into a healthy raspberry plant." [21]

Why can't we also use specific frequencies to change and heal our own Energetic Matrix?

This information is being researched in one sector of science, and yet is unavailable to us in western medicine.

Chapter 9

Structured Water and the GDV (Gas Discharge Visualization Device)

As time went on, all of this knowledge percolated in me. I had wondered about a new possibility. I had thoughts and glimmers of putting this all together. The general idea was there, but I didn't act on it at that time; I still didn't "get" the far-reaching possibilities I was to see and experience later. Early on in homeopathy, I understood water had some kind of memory, but the actual experimentation with this new form, what I now call "HeartFusion™," only happened in Ojai, California where I was inspired to experiment with it in a workshop I led.

This leap occurred to me after the last amazing pieces of information were revealed. Now I see it was so obvious; but then I just had a sense about it. It was waiting for the next part of my life to unfold! First it was homeopathy, then Emoto, and after that came information on structured water and ways to structure it with Clayton Nolte and the Russian Dr. Korotkov's GDV (gas discharge visualization device) .

These last pieces of the puzzle came quite a number of years after Emoto's information, when I met Clayton Nolte. Clayton is one of those amazing men you don't meet every day. He is a mountain of a man with a dry sense of humor. He likes to tease, provoke, and only supplies information when you pose a question; otherwise, he doesn't offer much. When he retired from his scientific job of forty years, he decided to dedicate himself to creating a better world with the knowledge he acquired working for someone else. In particular, this had to do with creating "structured water." He taught me about some of his discoveries, and also what Viktor Schauberger, a genius Austrian scientist (1885–1958), wrote about in the 1940s. You can read about Schauberger in a well-known book by Olof Alexandersson, *Living Water--Viktor Schauberger and the Secrets of Natural Energy* (1990). And *Hidden Nature: The Startling Insights of Viktor Schauberger,* by Alick Bartholomew, and David Bellamy (November 20, 2003).[22]

Clayton explained that living water, which is structured water, is found in icosahedral clusters. The hexagonal crystalline shape occurs when it is frozen. In its original natural state, it comes down the mountain stream or rivers, tumbling and whirling over rocks, and rushing over natural bends and curves (not in straight lines like pipes). That activity and constant motion "structures" the water (the structure we see in Emoto's photographs). In fact, constant motion is required to keep that water structured and able to "fulfill" the purpose for which it was created--to cleanse and nourish the environment. If it stops moving, it "dies," i.e., loses its life force which is then reflected in the loss of the crystalline form (only visible in ice). That structuring is necessary in order to support all of life. It erases the previous memory of frequencies harmful to life, and cleans and revives the water.

An interesting thought is that rivers and streams, as well as oceans, are "potentizing" or "succussing" the water with all of its minerals, and other constituents, through the very activity of movement--pounding over rocks, whirlpools, and the crashing of waves! They contain the original and primal homeopathic remedies made by nature, long before Hahnemann!

Nature is organized and coherent in its natural state, expressing what is called "Sacred Geometry" everywhere. "Sacred Geometry" is the term used for the repetitive basic geometric forms (based on mathematical codes) that always manifest throughout nature and the Universe, and as seen in Emoto's photographs (of course it is in 3D, but we see it as flat).

Since water imprints so easily, it picks up all kinds of energies and substances in its travels. This fact is both enlightening (as we will see in our work) and also disturbing in our polluted environment. These days we have heavy metals, all sorts of chemicals, and prescription drug residues that are now seeping deeper into our aquifers and more superficial underground water supplies. Some communities, needing more water, are now "recycling" their sewage. The frequencies and chemicals of Prozac, estrogen, fertilizers, herbicides, insecticides, hair dyes, paints, and an endless number of drugs and chemicals we all use daily, are becoming a nightmarish hodgepodge in our drinking water. The problem is not only on a physical level, but also on an energetic level of frequency. This pollution contaminates our drinking water in a profound way; as Emoto has shown, even the natural crystalline structure is destroyed. *It is a BIGGER problem than almost anyone understands.* So the value of structured water starts to emerge. Please remember, this information is controversial to those who do not understand energy. A chemist will not relate to what a quantum physicist understands.

Here is another interesting thing that Clay said--the "restructuring process" makes the harmful elements no longer available to the body, even if they continue to be in the water, they are drawn into the center of the molecule and washed out of the body. That is the way water cleanses your body, too, as it moves through you. When water is structured, it only promotes life and cleanses. The GDV images you will see soon show that water is capable of transmitting a very different kind of information to living matter. Farmers are seeing the results of structured water in their fields now. And, in one case, an organic dairy farm discovered that the very act of structuring the cows' drinking water actually eradicated the staphylococcus (an anaerobic bacteria) in their water. This is because the water becomes aerobic when structured.[23]

For the purposes of my research into HeartFusion™, homeopathy, and personal consultations, I use only structured water. This removes any chance that other energies will affect our imprinting process. If you don't have structured water (see Appendix 4 for information on how to get a water structuring unit), please use the purest water you have--filtered, reverse osmosis or distilled. As for your drinking water, you want to add minerals if you do drink reverse osmosis or distilled water because that water has none; it also is totally dead in terms of energy and photons if it is not structured. For the process about to be described, I prefer not to use bottled water in plastic because the plastic gives off its own estrogen-mimicking chemicals, among others. You DON'T want chlorine or worse, fluoride (a class 1 poison) in the water you use or drink.

However ultimately, when making your own HeartFusion™, if you have no choice and if all else fails, try whatever you have!

Measuring Structured Water with the GDV: (Gas Discharge Visualization Device) More Proof About Biophotons From the Russian "International Institute of Biophysics"

A few of us went with Clayton to Dr. Korotkov's seminar in Santa Fe in 2009. Dr. Korotkov's invention is an amazing computerized device that works like "kirilian photography on steroids," as he likes to say, called the GDV (gas discharge visualization device, see www.korotkov.org). He developed it in Russia. You can see everything that is off-balance with the emotions, the physical body and in the chakras (energy centers) using only fingerprints. It is different, but similar, to the results of Emoto's work, in that you can also see the effects before and after of thoughts projected onto water, or even into the energy of a room, using the GDV with special attachments. The computer program assists in the interpretation of the patterns of energy seen. In Russia they often use this tool for medical diagnostics! The GDV makes visible the energetic patterns that are given off by the photons in any substance--animal, liquid or solid. It is plain that water has no energy (i.e. photons giving off light) in the form of tap, distilled, or reverse osmosis water. With structured water from one of Clay's units, or from a natural moving body of water, there is a big difference! See the GDV photos:

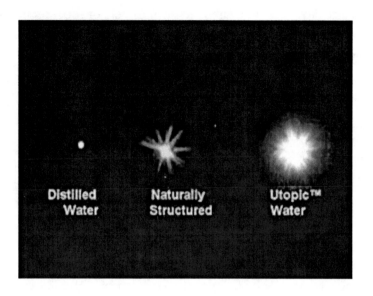

Distilled Water   Naturally Structured   Utopic™ Water

See http://www.utopicwater.com/research.html

The GDV unit can measure the electro-magnetic field of discharged biophotons (light energy emitted from a person or a substance). Utilizing this tool, research confirmed that good water from a Taos, New Mexico, deep well put out 15% bio-photons, more than you would expect from most other sources. After being run through Clayton's device, a tubular shaped unit housing internal geometric patterns, the water was re-tested. The biophoton discharge from the water dramatically changed to 87% bio-photons (light energy). The water became much softer and hydrated the body much better than unstructured water. The tap water we now drink is dead water. Water, even structured water, will lose its structuring and aliveness when stationary in bottles (unless they are cobalt blue), or when run through straight pipes of 300 feet or more.

Dr. Korotkov has appeared in a number of documentaries, including "Water: the Great Mystery," along with Dr. Masaru Emoto. You can view the movie here:
http://topdocumentaryfilms.com/water-great-mystery/
or see it on YouTube:
http://www.youtube.com/watch?v=s2Yn4AEWXD4
or order it from David Sereda.[24] I highly recommend it!

Biophotons are very weak pulses of light, but their "weakness" does not imply that they are weak in their effects. "We know today that man, essentially, is a being of light….and the modern science of photobiology … is presently proving this. In terms of healing, the implications are immense. We now know, for example…that genetic cellular damage can be virtually repaired, within hours, by faint beams of light…." Dr. Fritz Albert Popp. This is quoted in many places, but I was not able to find the original source. At http://www.viewzone.com/dnax.html it is said he said it in an old documentary.

In a later experiment, Dr. Samuel Berne, alternative optometrist who also uses a GDV, attended one of my workshops in Santa Fe. He kindly offered to measure the effects of my new technology before and after. While this turned out to be more challenging than we had envisioned for many tactical reasons, the results did show changes before and after HeartFusion™ sprays were employed.

More recently Annette Deyhle, PhD, Research Coordinator, Institute of HeartMath, Boulder Creek, California, was able to track immediate changes from incoherence to coherence after using the HeartFusion™ Spray. As she said, "This amazing technology quickly shifts a person from a stressful and incoherent experience into a state of coherence and balance. I personally experienced her simple and efficient approach, while monitoring myself with the em-Wave desktop (from the Institute of HeartMath) and I immediately achieved a state of coherence and inner peace after using my custom-made essence."

In the Santa Fe workshop with Dr. Korotkov, we did an experiment and measured the energy in our seminar room before and after a meditation: it was dramatically different! It was fascinating to hear about the development and uses of the GDV. Krishna Madappa, from Taos, New Mexico, is a colleague of Korotkov's and has been using the GDV for many years. He sponsored the event and has also been doing much research with the GDV. One such experiment was in a high school where he had the students focus on a drop of water; he then took GDV pictures of the drop. Then he had them project anger onto the water and he took more pictures. The difference is seen below.

This is the baseline of the water:

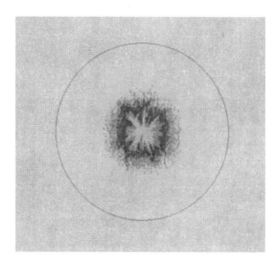

And this is a GDV photo of water that the class focused angry thoughts on:

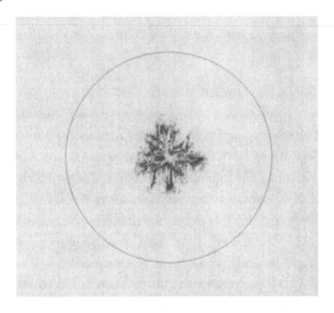

This is a GDV photo of water that the class focused loving thoughts to:

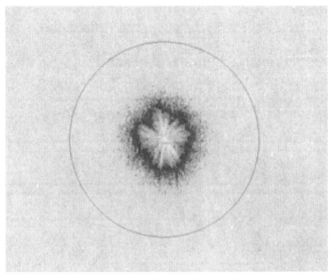

It is clear that the thoughts changed the pattern of energy of the water, as our thoughts do too every day!

If our drinking water is not structured, the water in our body isn't completely structured either. If you add a little structured water to a glass, the whole glass of water will be structured! The molecules automatically communicate with each other. Since we are made up of 70% water, putting *structured* water into our body seems more and more important. There are many devices that use magnets and/or electricity to change water. After learning about homeopathic imponderabelia (remedies made from pure energy), I think you will understand why those should be avoided--it is putting another unwanted frequency, with its own ramifications, into our water and therefore into our bodies.

Water has been used as a medium for baptism and many rituals from time immemorial. Only through the brilliant work of Dr. Schauburger, Dr. Samuel Hahnemann, Dr. Bach, Dr. Emoto, Dr. Konstantin Korotkov, Dr. Rustum Roy, Clayton Nolte, and many others in the field of water and energy, have we begun to see and appreciate the true essence of water. We have now been given some clues, enough to ask: How can we work with water to change ourselves and to change our world? Hopefully it's not too late. Everything that western civilization is doing destroys our water; we remove its life force and therefore our own. One hope is to restructure it, bringing it back to its original power and purpose.

So all together, homeopathy, research into frequency, Dr. Emoto's work, and information about structured water brought me to this new method for our collective wellbeing.

Chapter 10

Water, Essences and Frequency

Early Personal Experiences

I was perfectly happy to perceive the world through my "homeopathic eyes," it had become quite a habit! Then something different happened. I heard that a couple and their white buffalo, had moved to Flagstaff, Arizona. Being so near, I decided to visit them. The pregnant female white buffalo, Miracle Moon, was not an albino, not a "beefalo," but her DNA tested out as pure 100% buffalo. This was the first DNA-tested white buffalo. There were a number of new provings for animal milks at that time in homeopathy, and I was convinced this would make one amazing remedy! I planned to make one with her milk. I went up to Flagstaff to visit Jim and Dena Riley (see http://www.sacredwhitebuffalo.com and http://www.sacredworldpeacealliance.com) to ask if they would save me some milk after the baby was born. When I explained my mission they looked at me like I was crazy. "Ma'am, these are wild animals," Jim said. "We don't milk our buffalo!" I was crushed; for consolation, they offered me a piece of the fur Miracle Moon had shed. I was disappointed at first, but as I held the fur, my hand started to heat up and pulsate in a very unusual way. Immediately I realized the fur was something very special. I knew I needed to have a remedy made from it!

The Story of the White Buffalo

There are a few different versions of this story as you might imagine, because it has been handed down verbally over the generations; I will tell you the one I was told.

There was a time 1000 years ago or more when the Lakota people were in trouble. They could not find buffalo for the winter. They were cold, hungry, and there was much strife in the tribe as well as with their neighbors. Winter was fast approaching. One day two hunters went out looking for buffalo. Suddenly, in the distance, they saw a beautiful woman approaching. As she came closer, the first hunter was filled with desire and said he was going after her. The second tried to dissuade him, he also sensed there was something very unusual about this woman; but the first one took off, running towards her. Immediately, when he got near her, a mini dirt twister enveloped them both. When it stopped, the woman was standing there with a pile of ashes at her feet. The second hunter was scared, fearing he was next. She looked at him saying "This man had many desires and they were all fulfilled in a few moments, and this is what was left. You recognized me for who I am. Take me to your village and I will help your people."

During her stay, she taught the people to live in peace and harmony, and she gave them five ceremonies. The two best-known to us are the Sweat Lodge, and the Pipe Ceremony--

both incorporate the gathering of individuals to share their hearts, their truths and their prayers.

At the end of her teachings, she announced her departure. They asked when she would return again. Her answer was simple: "When the earth is in darkness and chaos I will return in the form of a White Buffalo to show the world there is still hope." She then walked off and led them to a herd to hunt.

In the process, she turned into a buffalo and her colors went from black to brown to red to yellow to white to represent all nations on the earth. Then she disappeared. Some Elders say she came from the Star Nations, or the Pleiades. The Pipe is said to still be within the Lakota Tribe.

See the White Buffalo and an interview with Jana about the essences on:

http://www.blip.tv/file/1988140

At present the Buffalo are living in Bend, Oregon, and are protected by a non profit organization.

See http://www.sacredworldpeacechurch.com/home.html and http://www.sacredwhitebuffalo.org or com.

The White Buffalo Remedy/Essence

So, as I said, being left with this special fur, I decided to invest in having it made into a homeopathic remedy. This process, of making a remedy from fur, being insoluble, is very time-consuming. Homeopathic remedies are usually made in special homeopathic pharmacies (supervised and approved by the

FDA), most of them are made by machines these days. It was an expensive process, but for some reason I felt driven to do it.

This was a time when I personally was going through a painful divorce after 19 years of marriage; I could see it was destined to be, but the process had ripped me up and triggered very deep issues. Finally I found a remedy for myself that had been recently "proven." It took a long time for me to come across this because it was a new remedy and I had very little knowledge about it. It was another Godsend in my life and removed the deep, physical ache that had been in my heart for the two years before and after the divorce. I was so relieved and grateful. But even with the new release I was experiencing, there was no strong sense of *joie de vivre;* joy was still not a part of my everyday experience.

The remedy arrived and I fortunately decided to wait until the workday was over before I tried it. My plan was to get quiet, meditate a little, and then take the remedy and see if I could feel its effects. A friend arrived that evening for some help with her neck pain. I asked if she would like to be a part of my experiment and be one of the two first people on the face of the earth to try this new remedy in order to see what it would do. She agreed.

We sat down on the couch and got very quiet to just to get a feel for where we were at, energetically and emotionally. Then we both took the remedy. As we sat there we both started to feel an expansion and a great opening of love in our hearts. There was a deep sense of gratitude and sacredness that we experienced. Even afterwards we both felt a deep joy that welled up from the inside… the effects lasted for a few days.

Of course I was so happy and grateful to feel love and joy again; but being the homeopathic researcher I was, I still wanted to see what this "proving" would be like. So I continued to take the remedy over the next few months in all the potencies I had ordered. Still, each time I took it I felt a profound sense of joy, gratitude and expansion. There was one point when I felt I was in constant communion with everything--not as if I were altered in a drug sort of way, but just feeling quietly aware. I had always wanted to feel that. At times, I felt as if I were in sacred prayer and union all day while working. I was so grateful for the experiences. I cannot say that those particular amazing spiritual states lasted indefinitely; however, the effects at that time were profound, and more than welcome. And to this day, whenever I use the Essence I later made, I feel the warmth and the joy again move into my heart. A that time it definitely moved me out of my stuck sadness!

One night I went to a party and saw a woman, Jeannie Michaels, whom I had treated years before. She took one look at me and said "I don't know what you are doing for yourself, but whatever it is--I want some!" I told her I had found something amazing, and took out the bottle of the remedy. It turned out her Dutch husband, Dr. Jaap Van Etten, is a very intuitive scientist who sees energy and auras. She led me to him and asked him to tune into the bottle. He looked skeptical but held the unmarked bottle; suddenly he looked very surprised and said, "Let's get together to explore this further!" I didn't tell them what it was until after we had had our first meditation together. In the end we meditated weekly for several years to research this new frequency and its potencies.

While Jaap, Jeannie and I continued to meditate every week, Jaap reported the information he was seeing energetically, and we all shared our experiences with the White Buffalo Essence. I was amazed to feel the same profound effects each week of love and gratitude. I was puzzled; how was "like cures like" manifesting with this? It was not behaving like a homeopathic remedy, not creating a group of "symptoms" that one would want to cure. Although this research was taking me in a different direction, I learned years later that Dr. Alize Timmerman in Holland (to whom I had also given the remedy) used it successfully in a homeopathic way with two patients. Both had reported a strong affinity to Buffalos before receiving the remedy.

When Is a Homeopathic Remedy Not Functioning in a Homeopathic (Like Curing Like) Way and Why?

In my quest to understand what was happening I shared this remedy with many people, individually and in larger groups of up to 40 in the form of a spray. Everyone felt similar effects. Finally, Alize Timmerman invited me to an international homeopathic conference in Holland where we experimented with the class. We actually spent an hour a day for five days grinding (we call it "triturating") the fur in a milk sugar base (no one else knew what it was) in the way insoluble substances are made into remedies. Everyone recorded their feelings, impressions and experiences over those days, which I have compiled (this is what we call a "proving"). No one but Alize and I knew it was from the White Buffalo. While there were a few people who had runny noses and mild symptoms during the proving, the majority experienced gratitude, love, a sense of the sacred, and expansion. There was also the desire to be physically closer to everyone in the room. In fact, for the first few days we all sat in groups of seven to ten in four separate groupings of tables; but one day one group emphatically insisted that we move all the tables into one big table. It was like bringing the "herd" together! Another day, Alize herself wanted us all to go and see an art exhibition that related to one of the topics during the conference. She marched our whole group in a herd-like manner for about 20 minutes through the streets of The Hague to see the outdoor event.

During this time, several students reported they had uncharacteristically shared deep personal information with total strangers. One homeopath, a very traditional Muslim, told me his large extended family always stayed in touch via phone and Internet; everyone was consulted on all matters relating to everyone. "You know though," he mused, "One thing we never discuss is our feelings." He later reported to me that after he had experienced the White Buffalo remedy, he had started speaking of his deeper feelings with his family, and soon they all started to do the same. It changed the whole family dynamics.

As far as I could see, this did not seem to be working "homeopathically," unless this remedy addresses a universal level of disconnection and suffering. When you think of how the buffalo were totally massacred by the white man, that may be a possibility. I still wonder....Another perspective is that this is such a harmonious frequency that it works in a very different way, simply resonating with our own internal harmonious frequencies. I haven't figured out the ultimate answer yet.

After discovering this White Buffalo Remedy, I decided to share it with more people. I turned it into an Essence (a milder version) and put it in a spray bottle. I have discovered that spraying a frequency into the aura (energetic field) around the body is very powerful. I really like that delivery system. I continued to use it in groups during meditations, and classes where we explored the power of vibration on consciousness. Everyone felt it. We also discovered its physical healing potential, especially on extremities. One friend with a broken little toe got total pain relief when we sprayed her from toe to knee both front and back of her leg. Since then, I have used it with people with numbness and pain in their limbs (even with post-polio syndrome or on diabetics) with great success.

So that is how I was led to Essences. I started to make others in different ways from very unusual sources that seemed to just "fall into my lap," and continued to research them, even while I continued my regular homeopathic pursuits. These HeartFusion™ Essences, as I call them, have been made from skin from frolicking whales (a deep sea diver captured it while it floated by him in Tonga), the energies of unusual crystals, and many others. All these were researched on people who sat quietly and observed what they felt before and after being sprayed. This is part of how I came to the idea and process, which I am about to share with you. So far, it is the culmination of my life experiences and knowledge.

The following are some captured images from the GDV made from two different HeartFusion™ Essences. This shows each HeartFusion™ has its own pattern and frequency.

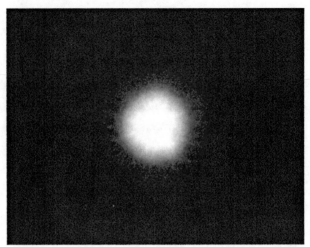

Protection

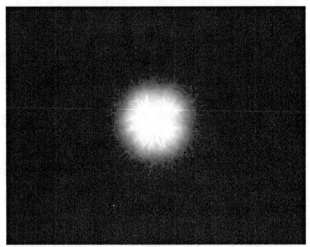

Unity

Of particular interest is these HeartFusion™ Essences are made not from a substance, like the White Buffalo fur and milk, but from a pure frequency and sensation transmitted into the water and then photographed. Although I do not have access at this time to the photo from another experiment we did, the GDV captured a picture of a HeartFusion™ Essence imprinted in water from the pain of separation and feeling of abandonment; it showed a whole ball of light divided in half!

A new book out called "Blinded By Science" (http://www.blindedbyscience.co.uk) by former skeptic Michael Silverstone is another great explanation about frequency, vibration and homeopathy.

Chapter 11

"C'est La Teraine!" "It's the Terrain!"

Today, medicine is based on the germ theory of Louis Pasteur. Interestingly, there was another brilliant Doctor of Science, Medicine, and Professor of Chemistry, Physics, and Toxicology whose name has been removed from medical history books. His name was Antoine Bechamp. He and Pasteur engaged in a life-long dispute. Pasteur claimed disease was only the result of bacteria attacking the physical body, and western medicine has embraced this theory.

Bechamp, however, claimed the "terrain," or the overall condition of the body, was responsible for whether tiny organisms called "microzymes" would change into a harmful bacteria or viruses which would then result in disease. The theory of "Pleomorphism" says when our body is out of balance on any level, the terrain changes; this allows for these "microzymes" to transform into what we would call "harmful" ones. They are then able to affect our body in the form of viruses, bacteria or even cancerous cells. Why does one person "get" a strep infection, or the flu, or pneumonia, and another not? It totally depends on the state of the person--or the host. Pasteur himself recanted his beliefs in his private journal, writing the famous words that were only revealed many decades after his death: "It is not the germ that causes disease but the terrain in which the germ is found" or, as it was reported he announced on his deathbed: "C'est la terrain!" Unfortunately, modern medicine does not even recognize the importance of this perspective, even though lip service has been paid to the effects of stress on the body. For a more detailed account see:

http://thehealthadvantage.com/biologicalterrain.html[25]

In classical homeopathy, we put a lot of emphasis on understanding the emotional terrain, requiring that it be taken into account and even brought to the forefront of understanding as a necessary requirement for all true healing. To understand or explain one level, we must always look to the next "higher" one; i.e. to explain water turning into steam we have to move to the level of atoms and how they respond to heat. I would say in many cases the mental and emotional levels are the "higher" levels. Bringing balance to those often allows everything else to come into balance.

In any case, what I am saying here is that instead of trying to *only* change the physical reality with medicines or even with the mind using affirmations and visualization, why not also change the total deepest terrain, i.e., the Energetic Matrix, to effect a deep cure so the individual will not be a good host to that bacteria or condition in the first place? I have not had the resources or the opportunity to apply this new technique to doing more in-depth research with what we would call physical "diseases." However, in more than a few people, physical changes have occurred. I would love an opportunity to research this more. As I have pointed out, in classical homeopathy we do this all the time. Some of the examples of physical changes occurring with this method will be mentioned here in the testimonial section. I look forward to hearing from you, my readers, to continue to learn more about this process.

Chapter 12
The Method, and Catching the Tiger by the Tail!

How it Came About and More

So now we stand on the very edge--the precipice--of a big dive based on so much amazing information and experience that is not a part of the "materialist mainstream" in medicine, or even many parts of scientific thought! Yet the steps, rough as some would imagine, are actually there...steps that have indirectly been acknowledged by some of the greatest minds on our planet. We are following the path that is beyond chemistry and Newtonian physics. If you are reading this book, you have already dipped your feet into this matrix, this Reality.

An Overview

This method, which was loosely rattling around in me for a while, coalesced one fateful day. I was about to give a workshop in April 2009 in Ojai, while visiting my healer friend Kenyon Taylor. I was tuning into what I should do with the group, when it became very clear: I needed to expand on the concept of "imponderabelia," letting each person make their own frequency for their own healing! It would be totally individual.

When the group met, I explained the following idea to them: we would go into a meditation. I would guide the group to connect with their deepest, most painful core issue that had a stranglehold on their lives. This issue always results in recurring patterns throughout life. Often, in the course of meditations I now lead in workshops or privately, people are surprised at what comes up, and new insights often surface. In private sessions, we can personally explore traumas together to determine the underlying core issue.

In the next step, I asked them to delve into this emotion all the way, feeling it as strongly as possible; ultimately it would become their most powerful medicine. When that emotion was established, I taught them how to capture it in water. I said "From now on, this tiger which has controlled your life will become your biggest ally! It is the best, most individualized, and deepest medicine for you! It now holds <u>your</u> power, <u>your</u> intention, and <u>your</u> truth. There is nothing stronger than that when used homeopathically; the power of your own frequency becomes your own medicine."

We imprinted the emotion into structured water, in cobalt blue one ounce spray bottles (cobalt blue best preserves frequency) and made a remedy from that imprint. Then, after making the remedy, we went back into the meditation, reconnecting with that emotion and the sensation it created in their body. Then we sprayed the remedy and observed the physical and emotional shifts that occurred. The results were dramatic for everyone!

Remember, your Energetic Matrix will know exactly what needs to be done to correct its imbalance! You don't need a middleman to effect a change! You do need to know the emotion behind the issue. You need intention and focus to proceed (as well as remembering to use your remedy later). Being in the energy of a workshop can be helpful. A personal guide can be very helpful, too; but ultimately it is *you* that will "take you home!" No one can literally do it for you. I am offering you nothing less than *a key to unlock your own empowerment*; it starts with the experience of an emotion and its corresponding sensations, followed by the imprinting of water.

Clustered Belief Systems: Finding the Core Issue(s)

In a workshop I recently facilitated, a participant said she wanted to focus on her desire to be loved. But after going through most of the process, she realized it was just an offshoot of a much deeper one: feeling totally unworthy of love, or "less than." She felt very small and unseen. The sensation and feeling of *that* was the imprint she needed; it was the true core issue that impacted everything else in her life.

Many experiences in early life ultimately lead us to an underlying belief, distortion, or as we call it in homeopathy--a "delusion." So it is important to be with our emotions consciously until we see through to the core issue, and *feel the core sensation, which is evoked by that emotion.* When I say "sensation," I literally mean the sensation in the body--the gut, the chest, the neck, wherever there is a shift in your body when you connect with your core issue. One question you might ask is, "What is the deepest most limiting belief or emotion in my life?" Or start with asking yourself, "What is the first memory of a traumatic event in my life and how did I feel in that moment?" Then observe how and if it reverberated throughout your life and experiences to come. You will always see that thread running through your whole life if it is truly a core issue! Often, working with someone one-on-one helps to uncover it more easily. Sometimes we can be blind to our most-obvious symptoms and clues. Over time we may also experience other emotions and sensations as they arise that we want to make into HeartFusion™ Essences too.

I have found, perhaps because of my training in homeopathic case taking, that it is usually easy to lead someone to that core issue and emotion which creates the same repetitive challenges over and over in life. Someone with a history of abuse, for example, will often attract abusive experiences with partners, friends, work relationships, and even other family members. Look at what pattern repeats again and again; then look for the emotion you feel that precedes it or accompanies it. The more core the issue, and the more tangibly we can experience it as a specific sensation in our body and Energetic Matrix, the better the imprint into water--the better the results. There can be multiple emotions relating to one incident. The important thing is to find one coherent sensation in the body. First connect with the core issue (like perhaps emotional pain behind anger), then be totally aware of the sensation rising up in your body, even if one word won't cover the feeling. One sensation is what is important. Then the imprinting will be successful. What you don't want to do is to mentally bring in another unrelated emotion, or worse yet, compile one emotion after another from your mind. You want to identify the *feeling with the total sensation* in the Energetic Matrix stemming from a core issue. If you come only from a mental, unemotional place, the imprint will be muddled.

One Example of a Pattern, the Sensation Behind it, and Changing the Neuropathways of the Brain

One client arrived with the pattern of starting projects with great enthusiasm and then "suddenly an energy comes in and whomp! I lose all ability and interest to continue. But," she said, "I cannot pinpoint the emotion related to the problem." I took her into a meditation and we revisited the first trauma she could remember. She had forgotten about it. It was a great moment of embarrassment when she was ten years old. She had been very popular in school and then one day in class she had to go to the bathroom really badly, but the teacher would not acknowledge her raised hand. Suddenly and uncontrollably her bladder gave way, and the kids saw her wetting the floor. She remembered the deep humiliation she felt and the sensation in her body of the shock, totally "freezing in horror." Everything stopped, and everything changed for her in that moment. She realized it was very much like the way her enthusiasm in life and with projects would suddenly come to a halt. She was teased by the same kids in that class from fourth grade all the way up to high school, becoming the scapegoat of her class. Then other memories flooded in about how other events leading to embarrassment had shut her down in her early life. We targeted that sensation--that feeling of humiliation that had her feeling frozen and shut down. Then she imprinted the water with that sensation of frozen terror. After finishing the potentization process, she sprayed herself with it. She felt an immediate shift in her energy and a great lightening of the continuous heaviness she had felt all of her life. This reaction is very common. Everyone seems to feel "lighter" and relieved of a burden or heaviness each time they spray the remedy (this may not register as very scientific in its description, but experientially it is very profound!). Some have said they feel like they are coming home to themselves--to their 'real' self underneath all of their "stuff." The process of sitting quietly in order to observe what is happening with the sensation before, during, and after using the remedy is very important. It is good to feel, and be imprinted with the feeling, of the unraveling process. As the new shift is repeatedly associated with the old imprints, new neuropathways of the brain are created which effect a more permanent change in the whole Energetic Matrix. This also includes the limbic brain and the cerebellum.

The advantage of being in a workshop is that the group energy is powerful in carrying us into the experience. Individual work, however, is much more personalized in targeting the specific emotion and sensation. In both situations, there is guidance with the imprinting and potentization process. Both experiences have their advantages. Just remember if you do work alone, give yourself plenty of time to be with each phase of this work, or you could miss out on something very important.

You Can Make a HeartFusion™ From Joy Too!

Until now, I have addressed working with the deep, challenging emotions that impact our lives. But surprisingly, I discovered this same process could be applied to the other side of the coin! Not only can we address the Law of "Like Cures Like" for our painful emotions, but we can also create HeartFusion™ Essences from the energies of love, joy and bliss, which we all want to experience in our lives; thereby activating the "Law of

Attraction" in a powerful new way! However, I feel that it is vitally important not to use the "positive" Essences just as a suppression or an escape. If there is emotional pain, use the positive remedy for joy *after* using the one made from the challenging emotion first. Often, a sense of relief and contentment follows after using the first remedy for the pain, and that opens into joy. The "joyous remedy" can be used afterwards, or just for the fun of it at any time, or during a meditation.

As we clear ourselves from the old emotions, we can turn to experiencing higher and higher frequencies. These can then be captured to share or re-connect with at a later time. Really, this is better than any artificial "high." It is legal, and will easily allow us to find those spaces at any time, and then move on from there. Taking this Fusion actually increases the power of your internal, coherent, harmonious frequencies. Your total Energetic Matrix will recognize it, accept it, and allow it to reverberate into the depths of your own being. This time it is *not* working in the "homeopathic" way of "like cures like." For the longest time I couldn't figure out why it didn't work in the same way as a homeopathic remedy. In other words, if two similar waves meet, they cancel each other out (just like those noise cancellation devices). If that is so, then why doesn't a "joy remedy" cancel out a "joyful feeling"?

This question nagged at me for months, then thanks to a discussion with a close friend, Franz Herbst, I realized that we always respond to any frequency when it is introduced. Then it is up to the *Energetic Matrix to act!* If it is a resonant, disharmonious frequency, it will trigger some type of self-corrective reaction. If it is a harmonious one, it will simply resonate and therefore be amplified within our Energetic Matrix. Basically we are not speaking of stimulus/response here (like one wave meeting with another and canceling the other out); we are speaking of:

stimulus/*organism* (i.e. *you*) /response!

That takes into account the self-corrective response from you! That is the big difference! Interestingly, I discovered my own (harmonious) joy remedy has had a positive effect on others too! If you meditate, you can also capture one of your beautiful meditations in the bottle to imprint and give back to yourself at another time when your mind is all over the place!. You can then start your meditation today from the energetic place that you left off once before! While part of the "work and exercise" of meditation is to still the mind, sometimes we just really need to be able to shift and slip into a peaceful, joyful place without the need of taking anything artificial to ourselves, like alcohol or drugs of any kind. It also offers an amazing opportunity to be able to share your energetic experience with others!

Chapter 13

How to Make Your Remedy, Step by Step: Creating Your Own Alchemy!

The Water

Here are the directions on exactly how to create your own alchemical remedy. Sitting next to us is a bottle (preferably a new spray bottle or very clean jar), filled with about an ounce of the purest water you have access to (structured if possible, if not, use filtered, reverse osmosis, distilled, or whatever water you have). As much as possible, avoid water with fluoride or chlorine. In making homeopathic remedies, structured water is ideal since there is no other memory, or other imprint, on it. In working with clients, I start with ideal conditions. If you cannot use structured water for your process, then proceed anyway, knowing that your emotional imprint will be strong enough to override the other chemicals and energies. Do this by mentally putting out the intention that the water be cleared of other energetics; that will help to structure it in its own way, too. Anyone can have structured water units in your home or office. You can check out Appendix 4 for more information.

The Bottle or Jar

Keep your bottle, spray bottle, or jar by your side. If you have nothing else, you can use a well-washed jar that doesn't smell of anything that was in it, including the dishwasher soap you may have used. Rinse it well in good water! You can also buy a dropper bottle or spray bottle in the cosmetic department of a health food store, large drugstore, or a store like Wal-Mart.

Directions: The Process

Put about three quarters of an ounce of water into a 1 ounce bottle, or if the jar is bigger, eyeball about an ounce. Homeopathic pharmacies have to be very specific, but for us it is not necessary. *Always leave a space between the water and the top of the container.* Now close your eyes, and go into a quiet internal space. If you are not familiar with meditation, please be sure to read the appendix on meditation. Just relax, and be aware of yourself--observe any tension in your body or agitation in your mind. Sitting in silence, begin to remember and feel an event in your childhood, or in your more recent life, that was painful, traumatic, fearful, or triggered anger, grief, abandonment, or some other strong emotion. Observe how event after event echoed that same issue or feeling throughout your life. Once identified, connect in with the situation(s) and run them through your mind over and over, allowing the emotion to build; all the while watching for your corresponding bodily sensations. Don't avoid any feelings. Really get into it! If necessary, revisit other similar instances. Feel it all--in every cell of your body, let it vibrate throughout! Cry if you want to! Let it take you over completely. The stronger you allow yourself to feel it, the better the imprint. This is your unique imprint! Your own brand of fear, terror, anger, abandonment, humiliation or grief--or whatever you are working with. Then, when the sensation of the feeling is very strong in your body, pick up your container of water and remove the cap; hold the bottom of the bottle or jar in your left palm and cover the top with your right palm facing downward toward the water (or if you are left handed you could try the reverse).

Visualize all the super charged emotion pouring through your hands into the water. If you are crying, you can even catch a tear in the bottle! You can even spit into it since your saliva carries the frequency, too! (It was found that saliva holds many chemicals related to the emotion present.[26]) Now hold that bottle for at least a few minutes, or as long as you feel like holding it, letting everything pour through you. You will know when you feel complete. Then put the top back on.

Succussion

Now, for the succussion part. This is critical. Make sure there is at least an air bubble in the jar or bottle. Hold the water in one hand and pound it really hard against the heel of your other hand 20 times. You can also pound it on a folded towel on a counter, or on the arm of a chair, or on the carpet. You should do it quickly and vigorously. Wimpy shaking won't work to make the HeartFusion™ remedy! Then empty the water, leaving only a tiny bit at the bottom, about an eighth to a quarter of an inch. Add more water, succuss again 20 times, empty again leaving a small amount on the bottom, add more water and shake again. Each time you add water and shake (succuss), you count it as one time, then two, etc. With each round you go up another potency. This cycle, always adding new water but *not* a new vibration, needs to be done at least 12 or 18 times; the more you do it the stronger effect it will have on you. I recommend, if needed, after 18, going up to 30 dilutions and successions, and then possibly more over time. It all depends on how often your core emotion will get triggered and how deep it may go; everyone is different.

After you make the remedy, sit down again in a quiet environment, if at all possible (one friend just locks herself in the bathroom to have some private space from her family!). Before spraying it or taking it, let your body calm down from all the shaking activity. Take some time to settle back into a quiet mode. Be aware of your body again. Reconnect with the tension, sensations and emotions you had with your core emotion. Once you reconnect with the sensation, *focus only on the awareness of your total Energetic Matrix and bodily sensations.* Use this as your meditation focus only, drop the story in your mind.

Be sure to feel where the sensation expresses in your body--do you feel fear, for example, in your gut, or tension in your chest, or somewhere else? Slowly scan your body from top to bottom, taking note of *what you are feeling and where.* Bring your full attention to sensing all the little nuances of pain, tension, and discomfort. Feel it in every possible way. Then, when you have a clear map of the sensations, and feel the emotion in your body, spray the remedy around your head, on the areas of sensation, over your chest, palms and heart center. Do this preferably on your bare skin. If you don't have a spray bottle, wet your hands with it and gently rub it all around as previously described, even put some in your mouth. Keep the rest of the remedy.

Then sit quietly and feel the shifts. Although you will feel something immediately, still give it a chance. If you can, ideally lie down or sit for 15-30 minutes, and feel the unwinding effects as they unfold. You will be surprised at what you feel. Continue to spray important spots of pain or tension as you wish during this time frame.

Now for your future use of this method, you don't *have* to sit quietly and feel the shift each and *every* time. You can spray it "on the go" if needed. However, it is really good to experience the "before and after" in your body and emotions, so you know how it is working with your Energetic Matrix. This is true particularly the first time you try a new potency. During this process your brain will be registering this new shift. One person described his experience as being so dramatic that even without stopping to pay attention, his awareness went from total fear and terror to suddenly feeling deep joy and gratitude with the first spray. It was replicated later each time he sprayed himself again. Sometimes it is just that dramatic! But if it is not so instantaneously dramatic, it is good to take the time to *feel* the shift. You will know without a shadow of a doubt that this process is working. Initially, everyone reports feeling lighter and more expansive; in addition, often deep insights and shifts also occur.

Occasionally, it may happen that your emotions feel more extreme after spraying; this is very rare, but the simple antidote to this is to make your HeartFusion™ remedy stronger immediately. Take it up as high as 30 succussion and dilution sets, and spray again. Everything will shift.

To Recap: This Technique Requires a Few Things for it to Work in Miraculous, Long-Term Ways

1. *That you become aware of your core issue and its related emotion and sensation.*

2. *That you catch yourself and are aware as that issue and emotion arises in your daily life. Some spiritual paths call this "mindfulness" or "self-awareness." After using your remedy, it becomes easier to do this, and your awareness increases.*

3. *That you remember to use your remedy consciously as soon as possible when the emotion, thought, and/or sensation recurs, or before an anticipated challenging situation. Keep it in your bag or pocket at all times.*

4. *If you no longer feel the beneficial effects, stop; realize that your Energetic Matrix is asking you to go to a deeper level in the unraveling process. Take the time to make it stronger by repeating the dilution and succussion process; then keep using it. Over time, keep increasing the potency if needed until you find the one that works well for you again. Don't give up! The number of dilutions you can make is only limited by your time and patience! Remember, homeopathic pharmacies have remedies that go up to 10,000 dilutions and more! If after increasing the potency a few times you still find it is not helping, it may be time to find a deeper core issue behind the one you have been working with.*

Again, this method allows your whole Energetic Matrix, to naturally self-correct, just like the Universe naturally self-corrects on every level in every moment. Our HeartFusion™ process is just what is needed to create the challenge for the

Energetic Matrix to jump-start into re-balancing itself that much faster. People say: "Time Heals." Well, "Time" does nothing! What happens over time is that the *Energetic Matrix has the opportunity to self-correct,* bringing you back into a more balanced state. This will make it possible for you to function, and ultimately function in a better way.

I sense there are many other possibilities for this imprinting process, as well as for the principle of "Like Cures Like." There is a potential to reach deep into many other spheres of life and different sciences. I ask you in other disciplines to please explore this with your creative minds; the Universe is alive, interactive, and constantly changing and responding! I challenge you in other areas of thought to consider how this phenomenon manifests in your field of expertise. There is much to explore and myriad uses, whether you examine "Like Cures Like" or the amplification of harmonious frequencies. Even in western medicine, drugs may be able to be more tailored to the individual. Low potencies made from chemicals found to be low in the body may stimulate the body to respond and rebalance itself.

The Additional Value of this Method: Increasing Objectivity and Awareness.

In contemplating this HeartFusion™ method, I have wondered whether this could go quite as deeply as a high quality, constitutional remedy for an individual. I think that is variable according to the person. This method definitely addresses *one* targeted issue at a time; if this turns out to be the *ultimate* issue, it may affect many levels. But for most, there are a combination of interrelating issues and symptoms. I am only in the early stages of this work. It will be interesting to see the effects with very high potency dilutions over time. Most people do not have the energy or patience to take the remedy into high dilutions like a 1,000 by hand! This potency is often what homeopaths use to change deep emotional patterns; but even if it were taken up slowly over time to a 200c, it would tell us a lot!

The beauty of this method is that it can serve us for the rest of our lives! All you need is water and a bottle or a jar. What if there were no homeopaths, or no access to drugs, remedies or herbs because of a financial problem or a natural disaster? In using this method, dealing with core issues that severely limit our lives, we foster a greater awareness of ourselves, our emotions, and how they affect our perception of "reality." We also eliminate our sense of helplessness, because we are now empowered with a tool to change ourselves.

Another positive aspect is that we come into a greater objective awareness of ourselves. In deeper terms, it brings us into the "observer" or the "witness" as it is called in some traditions. One patient called it a "double gift." You get the remedy and you get the ongoing awareness! She was shocked to see how often during the day she thought of herself as repulsive and unattractive! With this tool, you don't avoid or suppress your feelings, but you learn that there is someone else "in there" i.e. your own self, the observer, behind the part of you lost in the emotional whirlwind of delusions. The more your "cobwebs" of limiting beliefs and emotions dissolve, the more you can enjoy the real you behind it all! And you will be surprised at who that real you *is!* It is important to feel, but also important to realize that you go beyond just being a ball of emotions which come and go....behind them YOU ARE, as pure awareness.

Emotions are transient, YOUR CONSCIOUSNESS is not! You will begin to recognize the calm, centered, compassionate place that resides in the eye of any storm…your true self that is really YOU! In using your spray, you will easily come back to that place. At first, the important part is remembering to use it! That awareness will help in and of itself. Knowing you can return yourself to that place is almost as valuable as actually going there! In fact, you can train yourself with the spray to return to that centered place over and over. There will come a time when you will just do it because you will remember that space, and your brain's neuropathways will remember it too, it will become an automatic response triggered by awareness. So your HeartFusion™ not only helps to dissolve those places where you get stuck in the first place, but it also opens the door to see who you are behind it all! You can see how this whole process becomes an exercise towards growth, transformation and greater awareness! This is an experience that will evolve with you, not a suppressive one superimposed on you from the outside.

Now Is the Time

This is your time; this is your moment to allow for change and transformation. We all need it; the world needs it! If everyone on this planet could resolve their deep issues of pain, anger, fear and greed, how different everything would be! As each one becomes more free, it effects us all.

This HeartFusion™ process of contacting your pain may sound dramatic. It should. This deep re-visiting of your most-painful times, your deepest darkest fears, only need happen once for this remedy to be made and the healing to be deeply set into motion. I do not believe in dwelling on the past, but we all know how the effects of the past have colored our present lives. Our subconscious often attracts unhealthy situations and people to re-create our past, in a hopeless attempt at "fixing" it (or them) and making it right this time around! How many times have you found yourself in a situation, or a relationship, that was just like the previous (disastrous) one? Or one that is similar to one from your childhood? Unfortunately, any "fixing" never works. You cannot "fix" anyone out there. You can only change your own Energetic Matrix--that invisible field that exists within and around you. As Dr. Bruce Lipton has stated in his writings and lectures: "Thoughts *are* the energy field." Again, to reiterate, Einstein said "The field is the sole governing agency of the particle." We have to bring our subconscious thoughts into alignment with our conscious ones if we want to create a different reality from the one we presently inhabit. Interestingly, each one of us is the Particle, the Wave, and the Field too! Now we become aware of how we fit into quantum physics! And all this has a bearing on "The Law of Attraction."

As we change our thoughts and emotions, we also change the neuropathways in our brains. This allows for new patterns of thoughts and feelings to become automatic over time. Each time you spray yourself with your HeartFusion™, you are contributing to, and reinforcing, a new pathway in your brain. We know this must be true because when using the spray, emotional patterns change over time with no effort or resistance. Dr. Joe Dispenza[27] elaborates on this kind of change in his works and lectures. You can see a new pathway in the brain being formed on his website:

http://www.drjoedispenza.com/

Using Your New HeartFusion™ Remedy

Aside from the first time you experiment with your HeartFusion™ remedy, when you spray repeatedly a few times, I encourage you to generally use it up to two times a day if desired. However, in a crisis, use it as needed. Homeopathy is so different from western medicine because it is not, as I have already stated, suppressing symptoms, but instead stimulating your own healing reaction. If your emotions seem to get stronger, or not be touched as deeply as you wanted, take it up beyond the 12, to an 18 potency, or even to a 30. I have only had to do this on first making a remedy with a few people who have used this process.

I liken frequency of repetition to a car--you turn on the ignition and the car starts, if the car dies you turn the key on again. It is not very good to keep turning the key while the car is running-- the same way with remedies. You take them only when your "ignition" has died. With this method it may be tempting to actually take more because it feels so good. However remember how it sounds when you turn the key when it is unnecessary? Too many repetitions during each day may actually create a proving, so use only as needed--but do use it! Being a deep issue, you may want to take it once a day for a while. Even if the initial issue improves, be aware if the same pattern shows up under another guise.

For some, it will also be tempting to make all kinds of HeartFusion™ Essences, given what you now know. Be careful about mixing too many at once, as each one has a different set of frequencies. Keep it simple; make what you need. Ask your friends or spouse to remind you when to take it as you might forget in the heat of emotional upset. Also ask them to observe and report if they notice differences in you. They can see you better than you can see yourself.

Directions for Making a HeartFusion™ of Pure Joy and Bliss!

Get into a relaxed state, focus on the most wonderful, blissful, moments you can remember, or capture a wonderful feeling in the moment or during a meditation. Get into the complete sensation (past or present) and totally feel it in your body. When you have gone as totally as you can into those feelings and sensations, program your water by pouring that beautiful sensation, or all the love you could want for yourself, into that bottle. Then make a remedy in the same way described earlier-- by succussing and diluting six to twelve times. Usually the lower potency is enough. Then sit quietly and spray it on yourself and feel.

Using HeartFusion™ Essences with Children

We all know that children are incredibly creative and imaginative. They are also very deep and sensitive. I remember profound spiritual inner and outer experiences from childhood that I never told my parents about--and I loved them and we were very close. I just knew it was from my world and not theirs. I think a lot of us have had similar experiences. Yet as adults it is easy to forget a child's secret depth. At other times we may sense their emotion, but know it is inaccessible to us.

Children are excellent subjects for this method. Kids love magic, and this is like magic. They love the idea of having their very own "magic bottle" to use whenever they need it! They can even make the "positive" HeartFusion™, too, like self-confidence and joyous laughter! This process, this tool, can become a way to bond even more with your children, and support them with their deepest emotions. The great thing about using the HeartFusion™ method with your family is the process of communicating in greater depth about feelings, traumas, and the awareness of where and how they manifest. You will also be giving your children a method that can serve them throughout their lives.

Some children can really get into the whole process in a workshop. Some do better at home, making the remedy when the emotion arises. It all depends on the situation, and the child. A child with nightmares may do best having the process explained and then proceeding, with the support of their parents, at the time the bad dream occurs (if you can, succuss it once in the moment, then dilute it and succuss it again. You can return the next day to make the higher potency if this happens at an inconvenient time to do the whole process).

Another child may confess to a trauma or experience and be willing to participate in this process with you guiding them. But for those children who are more secretive, another tactic may work better. Giving them a bottle or jar and allowing them to do the actual imprinting alone in the privacy of their own room may work better. We have to respect the inner life of each child. After the imprinting occurs, you both can succuss and dilute the remedy together. A child has such powerful feelings and fresh emotions! Couple that with their ability to imagine and re-create emotional states...of pain or joy...and you have a great HeartFusion™! Think of the fun of creating a positive remedy from the joy and giggles of a child! And what a gift, for them to be able to instantly return to that same "space" again with a spray they made themselves. How nice to teach an alternative method for handling emotions and finding joy without drugs!

Chapter 14

Testimonials

In all the workshops I have taught so far, there are always individuals who are actively experiencing some sort of physical symptoms. I have heard people say "It is just stress." Well everything is somehow "just stress"; what is important is how YOU manifest that stress in your body. Some feel tension in their necks, others in their solar plexus, some get migraines, some get sore throats. When the core issue relating to that physical symptom is uncovered, there will be some kind of relief--sometimes very dramatic. It often comes when the remedy is sprayed directly on the physical center of pain; and don't be afraid to make it stronger if the pain only partially subsides. The remedy that cured my sciatic pain was a 50 dilution!

Release of Pain

It started in the first large workshop I led. One woman had a terrible knot in her back. She had been massaged, adjusted, acupunctured, given physical therapy, Rolfed, etc., and nothing had worked. She made her remedy, which was based on the feeling and sensation of constriction in her life. When she sprayed it on her back, the pain disappeared immediately! It was not enough that she had understood that the knot was related to her feeling constricted. Only when she sprayed the remedy onto the knot, could her full Energetic Matrix rebalance itself; the shift included the release of the knot, and the issue in her life.

Having been the child of a psychologist, and also having been in therapy in my younger years, I found it frustrating that after I thoroughly understood an issue, the related physical symptoms didn't disappear the way they were supposed to! Now I understand why: this is the next step I have been waiting for, for many, many years!

Trembling with the Memory of the Trauma

Another woman in one workshop obviously had experienced a very traumatic childhood. When we went into the emotional pain during the meditation her body shook and her leg jumped with muscular contractions. It was quite extreme. She cried quietly. After using the remedy she made with that pain, an amazing peace and joy came over her. I would say it was the most dramatic of anyone I had ever seen. When I checked in a few months later, a mutual friend told me she was still joyful and glowing, and still had been using the remedy.

Waking in Fright

Everyone to date has reported feeling lighter and brighter and relieved after spraying their HeartFusion™. I understand this is not enough to prove a scientific model, but I am relating this to you anyway. Several have called or written to tell me that whenever they wake at night and feel the gripping fear related to financial distress or some other fright, they spray themselves and everything releases and they can go back to sleep. We have not had enough time or support for an in-depth study of the progressive effects, as the potency is raised. However, from what I have seen with others and myself, I believe the potential is profound.

Panic Attacks in a Twelve Year Old Girl

I am so touched and deeply grateful to be able to share this beautiful story.

A woman who attended the workshop with her twelve-year-old daughter wrote:

"I believe my daughter had some kind of traumatic experience. I have no proof of what it might have been. She has either blocked it out or will not tell me about it. When she would go into panic attacks, she would hyperventilate and start tapping her hands very fast on her lap or some object. Her attacks used to be so bad she would feel nauseous too for quite some time afterwards. This has been going on for 2 years. The remedy she made for herself at your workshop started to work instantly within seconds! She has only had to use it 3 separate times. It used to be very hard to get her to calm down or even breathe, but when she used her remedy, it was instantaneous. She sprayed around her head and she was over it in seconds...quite amazing! Knowing that she has this remedy has empowered her. She has not needed it since we started, and it has been 10 months now!"

In fact she continues to report her daughter free of these episodes. It seems with her HeartFusion™ the previous "hard wiring" or neuroprogramming of her brain and Energetic Matrix self-corrected the imprint of the panic attack pattern. One can only imagine how this simple homemade remedy has changed this girl's life now, and has changed patterns that could have followed her for years to come!

Sciatic Pain Cured

Another close friend, massage therapist and homeopath with sciatic pain, wrote me after I guided her through this technique by phone:

"Please know that I am singing your praises in my heart for the brilliance you have now created. I am only on Day 5 and I have no gluteal or sciatic pain! My attitude, which is normally cheerful, is now buoyant and optimistic, and I am significantly happier inside. When I come home, I have sprayed an oral dose, as well as a topical spray on my sacrum, gluteal muscles and upper posterior thighs. Yesterday the pain was showing up in my mid-back (adrenal/kidney bilaterally), and upper thighs, which are symptoms that come occasionally, but today it is vanishing and there is just a shadow of pain! This is really a first! Thank you so very much!" Vero Beach, Florida.

Financial Fear

And another testimonial: "I was hit by emotional paralysis about finances. I sprayed my remedy for "unworthiness" during the day. A few days later, I increased the potency, as you suggested, six more times. Voila! It worked again and cleared the emotional heaviness and fear I was experiencing." K.W., Arizona.

A Letter from a Workshop Participant

"First, I want to share something very subtle that I've noticed in my years of benefiting from homeopathy. When pain leaves, we don't remember we ever had it. When I left your workshop, after making the HeartFusion™, I forgot there had been anything ever the matter! This has been especially true for me of your new breakthrough, a brilliant invention that allows us all to become our own healer by creating our own HeartFusion™. In my experience, I have found this process profoundly healing and transformative. We're all so used to things being difficult that it's even hard to believe that some deep seated, long standing emotional blockage or physical problem could exist for so long and then...be gone! Well, twice now, I've experienced the problems that I brought to the workshop dissolving after I took my HeartFusion™." S.Z. Sedona, Arizona.

And Another Letter

"Yes, I have my 2 remedies on my bedroom dresser and use them occasionally, every couple of days, or as needed or when the feeling strikes me. I feel that both remedies have made a difference. It's not that my behavior or outlook on the world changes drastically, but it's just enough to change what could be a negative attitude or a ho-hum middle of the road attitude, into an excited, upbeat "let's get this job done" feeling. One of them has to do with seeing/feeling BEING the JOY in life because I tend to be WAY too serious, way too much of the time!

The other was created for "Fear of Success," and it's clearly working! Over the years I could have been successful in half a dozen areas, but I got in my own way regularly. Now I just spray some "Fear of Success" around me and in my mouth, and barriers seem to melt away.

Thank you so much, Jana, for teaching this ability which we will carry with us for a lifetime!! Good Job!" A.N. Europe.

Feeling Alone After Divorce

"All my life I have had this deep fear of being alone. After my divorce, this feeling surfaced regularly. I would feel such a pain in my heart coming home to a house that was dark and empty. Somehow if there was someone there--even someone I no longer loved, it was easier. I never expected that. So I made a remedy from that deep painful, empty feeling. Wow! What a difference! As I would leave a party or a meeting I would spray it over my chest and belly and feel the tension and anxious knot dissolve. I keep working with it and making it stronger and it gets easier and easier. I have not even had to use it as much anymore. Thank you for this gift! Now I am going to make one for myself from my anger too!" J.H. Arizona.

After a Break Up

"I wanted to clear and heal the original separation I remembered. When I went back to my childhood and saw myself as a young child, I was watching my parents split up.

After spraying the remedy I made, I went from victim mode to thinking of that scene and saying: "What the heck are you doing!!!" I felt the sensation in my body shift dramatically. Then everything cleared and relaxed except my feelings about my most recent breakup. When I got home, I used it a few times and then was able to let go better. The next night I saw my old boyfriend at a party; ordinarily I would have been devastated; instead I went in the bathroom and sprayed my remedy, and it worked! I felt good, and very balanced in spite of it all!"

More Night Fears

"I awoke and lay in bed for a short time, turned on the lamp at 4:27 a.m., sprayed my "fear" remedy, went to the bathroom, returned to bed and sensed a calmness in my heart and heart chakra area with energy rippling outward into my energy field.

Another time I was having mid-month ovary pain/sensitivity. At 5:03 p.m., I sprayed the "joy/bliss" remedy. Pain stayed at same intensity. At 6:15 p.m. I sprayed my "fear" remedy and most of the pain and sensitivity diminished right away." L.D., Sedona, Arizona.

This is interesting, because if this had been the "placebo" effect, the first "bliss" remedy should have worked, but it didn't. In this case, it proved obvious the physical symptom was connected to her fear, and that is why that remedy worked for her.

A Core Issue: An Example of a Detailed Process from a Client Making a HeartFusion™

"After working with my main core emotion, I discovered another in another session. I remembered the first time I recalled feeling powerless. It was when I was three or four. My parents were sleeping later on the weekend and I was awake playing. Suddenly I saw what I now realize was a rat popping back and forth behind a radiator in our NYC apartment. It scared me--I had no idea what it was. I woke my parents to tell them there was something weird behind the radiator. In a groggy state they discounted my reality and went back to sleep. I knew it was real but they didn't believe me, and there appeared to be nothing I could do. I was not the kind of kid to scream and throw a tantrum, so I just felt powerless.

Tracing the feeling further along, I remembered experiencing that same frustration when I was taken to nursery school. I didn't like the teacher who sometimes hit us and then denied it when reported to my mother, at which point she got even nastier to me. I would decide at night that I absolutely would not go back there. I would be strong! But the morning would come and no amount of trying to convince my mother that I wasn't going back would work and off I got whisked to the nursery; powerless again.

I went over and over these experiences in my mind and the corresponding feeling, carefully observing the sensations in my body. I felt the hollow emptiness and weakness in my stomach and the shrinking of my being. I repeated the word "powerless" over and over. Then I picked up the bottle and held it open, with my palm facing downward over the orifice. I felt the energy of the sensation pouring down into my hands and into the bottle. Tears came so I actually let one roll into the bottle. I proceeded to make a remedy of an 18 potency from the frequency I had imparted. Then, still feeling the fullness of the emotion I sprayed it on me--my stomach, around my head, and in my mouth. Wow! It felt like every cell was drinking in the energy and feeling relief, I felt a tingling in and on my stomach. I let the reaction develop, watching the sensations in my body, for about 15 minutes, feeling the slow changes. Then I sprayed again twice more about 5-10 minutes apart. I felt a deepening shift each time. The next day I still felt filled up with a rare contentment. I felt happy to be alone and feel myself! My original remedy--related to a certain kind of feeling around abandonment, had a similar quality to it, but this had enough of a different flavor for it to still have a powerful and unique impact on me."

Again, what is important is to really get to ONE specific core sensation relating to a specific event, or a series of events with the same theme, and then really go into it so you feel it as strongly as possible in order to get a perfect imprint into the water.

Letter From a Homeopathic Client who had been Improving, But This Was Another Big Leap for Him

"Started the remedy I made of "insecurity." As you remember, my core issue had to do with my harsh father; I named it "under my own power; I count." I started the remedy on a daily basis five days ago. I had not noticed anything noteworthy until today. Yesterday I did not feel particularly good, even a bit queasy at times. At the end of the day, remarkably (given my lifelong chronic constipation), I had 6 evacuations! Then I had a dream at night:

"My father was upset with me for something--my not understanding well enough or quickly enough...that sort of thing. It felt so real, I felt my solar plexus so knotted up and contracting, I just wanted to shrink. Old stuff. But I 'moved on' at some point, finding someone I could communicate with so I could understand whatever it was I was not getting with my Dad. I woke up feeling really refreshed, cleaner, lighter, and more able. The point being, I was no longer stuck or frozen in time, and took action with no sense of the usual heavy, emotional baggage after the blockage with my Dad. Nice... A new change! Blessings and my gratitude." H. D., Denver Colorado.

Letter from a Woman With a Bladder Infection Whose Husband Had Committed Suicide

"I am doing really well. My bladder is definitely better, and I am going to the bathroom less frequently. Didn't take the 40 potency yet. But emotionally something is different. It's as if I don't have a 'charge' on my memories or the story of my former husband. It is very peaceful, like it all happened in another lifetime. And I *never* realized that I had a charge on the story when I was just going about my day (I knew there was a charge when I cried or something, but now I see the emotions were subtly there all other times too). I will keep you posted about the bladder. Feeling great regardless of what happens medically!" FS, Florida.

Anger

"The remedy I made from 'Powerlessness' really helped me through a situation where I was going to lose my mind, I was so mad at someone. It helped me to stay centered, and I felt much better with the spray!" BJ, California.

Rage

"My issue has been rage. I thought after all the years of therapy and different newer processes it was handled. But when you led us in the inner search for our core issue it popped up. I was surprised it was still there, only I did know I got angry easily with my partner. I just never associated it with that part of my past! I now see the other processes only put a Band-Aid on it. When I made the HeartFusion™ it blew me away--I felt the change the minute I sprayed it. Now I feel I have found a healthier path with the spray. I have a new awareness and a choice. When I start to feel the rage getting ready to click in now, two months later, all I have to do is think about the spray, and my emotions shift instantly. It is as if I have shifted somewhere else and now I can get back to that place by myself. It is getting to be less and less that I even go there. I can't thank you enough. I want all my friends to do this too!" TF, Arizona.

Not a Band Aid

"Making your own Alchemical HeartFusion™ is brilliant--and it worked permanently for me; I was the 'master stuffer' my whole life. I'll be more specific: my issues were 'unexpressed emotion and anger around Love.' It began in teenage years after an emotional trauma and I thought I was 'over it.' In exploring the deep cores of why I had manifested skin cancer, I had to dig deeper. You coached me through the process of making my own HeartFusion™ through Skype. I have not needed this 'remedy' since. I sprayed it on me after we worked, three separate times. Powerful work--and it is not a 'Band-Aid'...'patch cords' come to mind....In the old days of radio, you used patch cords to get the flow of energy from one piece of equipment to another. It is all about energy flowing out. I feel that this piece has been healed and it's been about 4 months.

"I've made others since--all with huge results and success! May you help as many people as possible. God Bless you and your work!" CJ, Denver, Colorado.

A Case of Terror--In a Woman, and Then Her Cat

A woman came in to see me and in her session the emotion of terror and helplessness came up. She had been born in a large family of 10 in an Asian country. She had been treated as "just a girl" and had been forced into an arranged marriage against her will. She had had a number of events that caused her fear in her early life. We identified them and made a remedy from the resulting emotions of fear and terror. The results were so dramatic I regretted not capturing them on video. She felt totally changed and reported a "new feeling" she could not even identify as she disconnected from the old ones. Two days later her affectionate cat went into a terror himself with no apparent cause, wailing and running and hiding. Not knowing what to do she grabbed her spray bottle and sprayed into the air around the cat (cats do not like to be sprayed). Instantaneously, the cat shifted, calming down and returning to his loving self, proving this can be used with animals too!

Chapter 15

In Conclusion

We have seen the power of the homeopathic principles; we have learned about frequency and water. We have seen the proof of energy and thoughts on water with Dr. Emoto's photographs and Dr. Korotkov's GDV.

So much is being written about the importance of reprogramming our thoughts and emotions so as to change our chemistry, and everyone is searching for effective techniques. There are wonderful books and movies that go into much greater depth on the subjects lightly touched in this book. Some of the movies are: "What the Bleep Do We Know?," "What the Bleep? Down the Rabbit Hole," and "The Secret." There are many incredible books like all of Gregg Bradon's. One of them is: *The Divine Matrix: Bridging Time, Space, Miracles, and Belief*,[28] and Bruce Lipton's books with scientific research relating to our thoughts and our DNA: *The Biology of Belief*,[29] and *Spontaneous Evolution: Our Positive Future*.[30] There is *The Power of Now*[31] by Eckart Tolle and of course, Lynne McTaggart's profoundly documented books, *The Field*[32] and *The Intention Experiment*.[33] There are many others that deeply probe these ideas. For a great book on different types of meditation and inner explorations, check out *Journey of Awakening*[34] by my first teacher, to whom I am eternally grateful, Ram Das. There are also techniques that are immensely helpful for many, like EFT (emotional freedom technique), EMDR (eye movement desensitivation and reprogramming), and NLP (Neurolinguistic Programming) to name a few. The combination of these methods and ideas with the HeartFusion™ method may make them all even more effective. The fact that in any moment you can grab your spray and instantly feel the amazing results is a big plus. Of course, challenges occur in our lives, but now we can make remedies from the emotions that get triggered, preventing them from making deeper and deeper grooves into what Eckarte Tolle calls the "pain body," or others call our "psyche."

The main purpose of this book has been to lead you into understanding a little about energies, frequencies, conscious awareness, and the basis of this method--a practical next step to changing your Energetic Matrix: "Your Field." I believe this alchemical technique is one of those gems, deceptively simple, and easy to use. We now see how it is possible to walk into your kitchen and create your own remedy to release suffering and reprogram your Energetic Matrix, dissolving the cords and neuropathways that bind you to it! Just as there is an ocean of tears and pain outside and within, so is there an ocean of Love waiting to for us as the pain patterns dissolve! This is a recipe for the transformation of body and mind, to support the soul! Give yourself this gift; you will unravel your "knots" more effortlessly than you think. Become a part of the ongoing inner evolution and revolution!

A Shift is coming, and as each one of us awakens within, so will others awaken too; we are all connected as quantum physics teaches. Look around. There is an urgent Calling--and the time is NOW!

Appendix 1

Laws of Cure

The following Laws of Cure are applicable to all forms of healing (western or other) except certain instantaneous energetic forms of spontaneous cure.

Hering's Laws of Cure says:

1. Symptoms go away from the deepest (most limiting) level to the most superficial

2. Symptoms resolve in the reverse order that they came: the most recent going away first

3. Symptoms should improve from above downwards.

4. Symptoms heal from the most important organ to the least important organ

5. Symptoms improve from the center of the body to the periphery.

Appendix 2

Isopathy: Making a Disease Remedy for Cure and Prevention

I want to explain about isopathy and how you can use it. As we have seen, anything soluble or energetic can be easily made into a remedy. Insoluble substances are much more difficult to convert unless you want to be grinding for 3-5 hours. There are homeopathic pharmacies that have machines to do that.

It is best to remember that when something is made into a remedy it may have different properties than the original substance. The lower the remedy potency the closer it is to the original substance and its uses. In potentizing a bacteria or virus, it is best to make a 12c or higher. At the end of the successions, you can add ¼ oz vodka if you want to be sure everything is "dead" that was in the bottle. Let it sit for 20 minutes. A drop to a teaspoon (remember as an energy the exact amount doesn't matter) can be taken 3-4 times for 1-3 days as needed. You can buy a one ounce bottle of vodka in a liquor store. If there is an ongoing epidemic, repeating it 2-3 times 1-2 days a week for a few weeks can work well. By making the remedy as described in this book, you can help yourself and your family!

Here's an example of isopathy: Many years ago a woman called me. She lived in another state. She had viral pneumonia. Antibiotics do not work on viruses, and the drugs her doctor gave her had not helped. She wanted a remedy. Although I knew the remedy after speaking to her, since it was Friday, an overnight package from a homeopathic pharmacy wouldn't arrive until Monday. So I made a suggestion, and told her to spit some phlegm into a clean jar, and then go through the process of shaking and diluting 30 different times (you could also stop at 12 times, but I wanted it to have a stronger effect because of the severity of her condition). I know this sounds awful, but as you do it, the water in the jar starts to look cleaner and cleaner. Thirty times is a lot! At the end, just to be sure and make her more comfortable, I had her add vodka and let it stand for 20 minutes ensuring that anything that might be left (which there couldn't be after so many dilutions) would be dead. Then I told her to take it every three hours. Within 12 hours she was doing much better, within two days she was completely well. We call this kind of remedy a "nosode"--one you make from a disease bacteria or virus. It isn't always as effective as something that is *similar* to the symptom picture, but sometimes it works like a charm! It's worth a try if you don't have access to any other form of treatment.

I also tell parents to make a nosode by swabbing the throat or nose with a Q Tip and swishing it in water when one person gets sick in the family. They can make it (similar to a vaccine) and give that remedy to the other family members a few times a day for 1-3 days to prevent the spread of the disease.

Appendix 3

Meditation for Those New to It

Since some of you may not be familiar with meditation, I want to include this important part. In our particular method, it is good if you use your powers of observation in a meditative way. I personally am a big advocate of meditation and it has been an integral part of my life since my early 20s. There are many ways to quiet the mind and turn down its volume so you can feel the part that is you behind all the mind chatter. Yes there is more of you--you are not just your mind. But without the opportunity to be aware of your non-mind essence, how would you know?

Short tips for meditation: Make no mistake--your mind WILL wander off, it is natural; as the Buddhists say--you tongue tastes, your eyes see, your nose smells, and your mind thinks. So don't get upset, but gently bring your awareness back to *one* of the suggested methods of focus below.

Techniques for focus and awareness include:

1. Total awareness of your body in the moment. What do you feel? What is tight? What feels good? And be aware of the part of you that is watching,

2. Total awareness of the moment--everything, and every energy around you.

3. Imagining breathing into your heart center in the upper middle of your chest. Visualize breathing a golden mist in and out of your chest.

4. Awareness of the breath coming in and out

5. Repeating a soothing sound (Like Aum) or a word over and over again; when the mind quiets, let go of the word or sound. When it starts up again, return to the repetition.

6. Focus on a picture of Christ, Buddha, or whomever you are drawn to, (or even focus on a candle). Breathe their light into your heart center.

Experiment with one of these methods; as your mind wanders to somewhere else gently return to the method of choice. Be patient, like with a child, bringing yourself back to the focus you have chosen. It could even be a scene on the beach while relaxing in the sun.

In general the important thing is to give your mind something to focus its attention on. The idea is to find a focus, or more than one, to occupy the mind. When you do that, and do it for a while, a sense of peace will come over you. Sometimes it can take 5 minutes, sometimes 45 minutes, but usually there will come a point of a major energetic shift; then you enter the "zone," and even if the thoughts continue to drift by, you will feel a place where you exist behind them. It is wonderful to begin to discover that part of yourself. Try it for 5, 10 or more minutes. Some days it will be easier than others, so don't get discouraged. You can certainly try it with one of your HeartFusion™ sprays.

<u>A Great Tip for Everyone</u>

If you have any trouble breathing or feeling your breath constricted, or if you have any lung-related problem, try this: in each hand hold the tip of your thumb to the tip of your ring finger. This opens the lower lobe of your lung, and automatic diaphragmatic breathing. If you include the tip of your middle finger too it also opens the middle lobe of your lung. This is a trick I learned from Dr. Lad in an Aryvedic workshop many years ago.

You may see pictures of yogis holding the index finger with the thumb tip--this reduces breath to the very top of the lung and is only used to induce shallow breathing and breathless states. This is not appropriate for our work.

Appendix 4

Structured Water

As mentioned, Clayton Nolte has developed convenient ways to make affordable structured water available to everyone. He has devised units for travel, for the shower (portable and screw in), for under the sink, and one to install for the whole house. These units are unique in that the structuring occurs through the movement of the water through a pattern of channels. There are no other moving parts, no use of electricity or magnets that will imprint water with their own frequency. This water is clear and without other memories. For more information check out his website at <u>ClaytonNolte.com</u>. For ordering information email <u>info@healthrays.com</u>. Also, you can visit my website <u>http://www.healthrays.com</u>.

Index

ADD / ADHD, 53

Bechamp, Antoine, 97

Children, 12, 53, 54, 59, 119, 120
Classical homeopathy, 26, 98
Core issue, vii, ix, 101, 102, 103, 113, 115, 122, 130, 132
Crystalline structure, 63, 64, 65, 79
Cuba, 58

Dispenza, Dr. Joe, 117

Emoto, Masaru, v, 63, 64, 65, 67, 77, 78, 79, 81, 83, 86, 134
Energetic Matrix, 25, 27, 28, 31, 32, 39, 40, 44, 45, 46, 48, 52, 61, 62, 75,
    76, 98, 102, 103, 105, 106, 111, 113, 117, 123, 125, 135
Essences, 87, 94

Frequency, ix, 25, 28, 33, 36, 56, 57, 64, 65, 67, 68, 70, 72, 75, 79, 86, 91,
    93, 94, 101, 106, 110, 118, 130, 134, 143

GDV, 77, 81, 82, 83, 84, 85, 134

Hahnemann, 20, 23, 24, 25, 79, 86
Homeopathy, viii, ix, x, 17, 20, 21, 22, 23, 26, 29, 31, 34, 35, 38, 39, 40,
    41, 52, 53, 54, 55, 56, 57, 58, 59, 60, 63, 64, 67, 72, 77, 80, 86, 87, 102,
    126, 146

Imponderabelia, 54, 55, 86, 101
Isopathy, 59, 60, 138, 139

Korotkov, Konstantin, 77, 81, 83, 84, 86, 134

Law of Similars, 23
Laws of Cure, 39, 41, 51, 137
Leptospirosis, 58, 59
Like Cures Like, 48, 92, 105, 106, 114

Mallon, John, 68, 69
Meditation, 14, 47, 50, 84, 91, 101, 104, 107, 109, 111, 123, 135, 140
MEG, 67

Citations

[1] http://www.slideshare.net/drprabhatlkw/homeopathy-in-pandemics-epidemics. Also see
http://www.homeopathy.inbaltimore.org/saine3.html

[2] Ibid.

[3] Czerlinsky.

[4] "The Homeopathic Revolution: Why Famous People and Cultural Heroes Choose Homeopathy" by Dana Ullman MPH and Peter Fisher MD North Atlantic Books, 2007

[5] See Sue Young's website:
http://homeopathy.wildfalcon.com/archives/2010/02/07/fewster-robert-horner-1803-1863/

[6] "The Science of Homeopathy" by George Vithoulkas. Athens A.S.O.H.M., 1978.

[7] http://hpathy.com/homeopathy-scientific-research/homeopathy-%E2%80%93-how-it-works-and-how-it-is-done-2/

[8] "Homeopathic Potencies Identified By A New Magnetic Resonance Method: Homeopathy--An Energetic Medicine" December 15, 2006 by Karin Lenger.

http://www.issseem.org/storejournals_detail.cfm?articleid=210

http://www.youtube.com/watch?v=O9g9dz1U0qA&feature=related with Dr. Glen Rein

http://www.heartmath.org/research/research-home/research-center-home.html

Czerlinski' and Ypma "The Water Journal" January 2010 "Domains of Water Molecules Provide Mechanisms of Potentization in Homeopathy" http://www.waterjournal.org/volume-2-index/63-czerlinski-full-text

[9] "The Message from Water" Masaru Emoto. Published/Created: Carlsbad, CA : Hay House, Inc., 2009.

[10] "The True Power of Water" Dr. Masaru Emoto Hillsboro, Ore. : Beyond Words Pub., c2005

[11] http://www.heartmath.org/faqs/research/research-faqs.html.

[12] John Mallon's website http://www.thehealinguniverse.com

[13] http://www.thehealinguniverse.com/library.html

[14] Video 3 on http://www.thehealinguniverse.com/videos.html

[15] http://www.thehealinguniverse.com/library.html "Russian DNA discoveries" Fosar & & Bludorf #34

[16] "The Secret Life of Plants," Peter Tompkins and Christopher Bird. Edition Information: [1st ed.] Published/Created: New York, Harper & Row [1973]

[17] http://www.thehealinguniverse.com/library.html [34] Fosar & Bludorf "Russian DNA Discoveries"

[18] http://www.bibliotecapleyades.net/ciencia/ciencia_genoma19.htm

[19] http://www.thehealinguniverse.com/library.html Fosar & Bludorf #32 "Recent DNA Discoveries" by von Barbel Mohr and "Russian DNA Discoveries" by Fosar and Bludorf #34

[20] http://www.thehealinguniverse.com/library.html Tom Beardon #33 "Extraordinary Biology"

[21] http://www.bibliotecapleyades.net/ciencia/ciencia_genoma19.htm

[22] "Living Water - Viktor Schauberger and the Secrets of Natural Energy" (1990). And "Hidden Nature: The Startling Insights of Viktor Schauberger" Alick Bartholomew, and David Bellamy (November 20, 2003).

[23] http://thebovine.wordpress.com/2009/09/01/structured-water-affects-bio-photons-eliminates-staph-bacteria-for-raw-dairy/

And http://www.naturalactionwater.com/

[24] http://www.voiceentertainment.net/litecommerce/cart.php?target=product&product_id=257&category_id=60

[25] http://thehealthadvantage.com/biologicalterrain.html

[26] "Your Cosmic Destiny" by W.A Chapman which is out of print. "The poison of a few minutes jealousy is enough to kill a guinea pig. An hour of hatred produces enough poison to kill 80 guinea pigs…"

[27] http://www.drjoedispenza.com/

[28] "The Divine Matrix: bridging time, space, miracles, and belief," Gregg Braden, Published/Created: Carlsbad, Calif., Hay House, 2007.

[29] "The Biology of Belief: unleashing the power of consciousness, matter & miracles," Bruce H. Lipton. Carlsbad, CA : Hay House, Inc., 2008.

[30] "Spontaneous Evolution: our positive future (and a way to get there from here)," Bruce H. Lipton and Steve Bhaerman. Carlsbad, Calif., Hay House, c2009.

[31] "The Power of Now: a guide to spiritual enlightenment," Eckhart Tolle. Novato, Calif., New World Library, 1999.

[32] "The Field: the quest for the secret force of the universe," Lynne McTaggart, 1st ed., New York, NY, HarperCollins, c2002.

[33] "The Intention Experiment: using your thoughts to change your life and the world," Lynne McTaggart, 1st Free Press trade pbk. ed., New York, Free Press, c2008.

[34] "Journey of Awakening: a meditator's guidebook," Ram Dass, edited by Daniel Goleman with Dwarkanath Bonner and Ram Dev (Dale Borglum); illustrated by Vincent Piazza, Rev. ed. New York, Bantam Books, 1990.

About the Author

Jana Shiloh, M.A. CCH, HMA, H.H.

Jana Shiloh received a Master's degree from The New School for Social Research. She has taught and been active in the homeopathic world for 30 years both nationally and internationally. She helped to found the Pacific Academy of Homeopathic Medicine school in 1989. In 1990 she was named "Honorary Homeopathic Clinical Associate" by Dr. Ronald Davey, the physician to the Queen of England. She taught homeopathy in a course taught at The University of Arizona Medical School in Tuscon, which was co-sponsored by Dr. Andrew Weil. She is nationally Certified in Classical Homeopathy and presently practices and teaches in Arizona as a "Hahnemannian Healer" (known in other states as a "homeopath"). Her HeartFusion™ Essences are a part of "Sedona Sacred Essences™," which also includes "White Buffalo Bliss™." Jana facilitates workshops, "Skype-shops," webinars, and private sessions, both in person and long distance. Her workshops and sessions are offered in Classical Homeopathy, The HeartFusion™ Method, and various ones based on her other Fusions Essences. She continues with her practice, and her research into water, frequency, consciousness, homeopathy, and health in Sedona Arizona.

Many Essences are available through her. See the following page or go to her website: Healthrays.com. She can be contacted at info@healthrays.com.

More Information About the Fusion Essences

The Evolving Line of Sedona Sacred Essences
Available Through: http://healthrays.com/

Watch the website for new entries.

White Buffalo Bliss™ (Female)
For opening the heart, for sharing with others, for couples to share together, for ceremony, for meditation, for expansion in consciousness, for gratitude, joy and love. This one is made from the fur and the milk of Miracle Moon when she was pregnant.

Sedona Healing Power with White Buffalo
A Spirit-Fusion combination to heal pain and injuries.

White Buffalo Crown Chakra (Male Fur)
A Spirit-Fusion for serious meditators. Must order in person by phone.

Whale Dreams™
For slow deep dives into the Ocean of Awareness.

Atlantis Rising™
A powerful energetic from an Atlantean artifact, for Serious meditators. Must order in person by phone.

Maha Avatar Kriya Babaji
Four Different Visitations: Aura Activation, Merging, Milk and Honey, and Blessings.

Platonic solids
Sacred geometry Essences starting with the triangle and going up through the Star Tetrahedon up to the 12 sided dodecahedron. Order individual ones or the whole set.

Lakshmi (Abundance Energy)
HeartFusion™ Spray to use with a meditation. MP3 meditation soon to be released on healthrays.com.

A full set of individual **Chakra Activators** 4-7, plus the first 3 together as the "foundation energy," order one or all of them. Made from the tonal sounds of Ashok Kumara. Other titles:

Sai Baba's Love	**Self Confidence**	**Bliss**
Q'uan Yin	**Union**	

Your own HeartFusion will be the most effective, but if you don't make your own:

For Insecurity (female);

For Insecurity (male);

Divine Love ;

Divine Mother;

Angelic Presence;

For Abandonment Issues;

For Contraction in the heart and solar plexus;

For Feelings of Lack of Support.

For Deep Grief;

For General Grief;

For Computer Sensitivities;

For Cell Phone Sensitivities;

For Solar Flare Sensitivities;

For Protection Surrounding You From Above;

Vedic Precious Gem Protectors (ask for the 1 you need).

Coming soon: powerful Vedic fire ceremony essences, & more!
Go to healthrays.com to order, or call 888-282-9362 (PST).

CPSIA information can be obtained at www.ICGtesting.com
Printed in the USA
BVOW01s1030240913

331692BV00004B/18/P